# LONDON'S EMERGENCY SERVICE VEHICLES

Dave Boulter

AMBERLEY

Front:
*Top*: Soon after daybreak on a Saturday morning, an emergency ambulance and Volvo estate head down Whitehall.

*Bottom*: A City of London Police BMW X5 and Ford Focus estate dog handler unit parked in the shade near St Paul's Cathedral in an 84-degree Fahrenheit heatwave; 30 seconds later the dog unit was to mobilise down Ludgate Hill on an emergency.

Rear:
The crew of Soho's turntable ladder in the process of making up equipment in Gerrard Street after a six-pump incident just 100 metres from the fire station.

First published 2017

Amberley Publishing
The Hill, Stroud,
Gloucestershire, GL5 4EP

www.amberley-books.com

ISBN: 978 1 4456 7193 2 (print)
ISBN: 978 1 4456 7194 9 (ebook)

British Library Cataloguing in Publication Data.
A catalogue record for this book is available from the British Library.

Typeset in 10pt on 13pt Celeste.
Origination by Amberley Publishing.
Printed in the UK.

# Contents

# Foreword

## Behind the Sound of Sirens

So busy is the central London emergency vehicle scene it is rare to wait more than a few minutes before once more the distant sound of sirens is heard, accompanied by the flicker of blue lights and glare of headlights appearing in the distance, often then swallowed up in dense traffic.

Whether your interest is police, fire, ambulance, or associated emergency and rescue services, this fully illustrated book of nearly 200 images captures central London's many 999 services going about their daily business. These are the vehicles behind the sound of sirens so often heard in media broadcasts coming from the Whitehall area.

Many of the images vividly capture fast-moving vehicle response on the blue light as emergency crews battle through London's congested streets. Crowds and congestion are the reality of central London and, deliberately, no attempt has been made to disguise that. Thus, the full authenticity of that precise moment in time is retained, allowing the reader to visualise themselves stood alongside the photographer as the images are captured.

## The Range of Organisations

Complementing vehicles from the London Fire Brigade, London Ambulance Service, London's Air Ambulance, London Fire Brigade and the Metropolitan Police Service are those of the British Transport Police, City of London Police, and Ministry of Defence Police. The Royal National Lifeboat Institution, British Red Cross Society and St John Ambulance are also included, as are the London Underground Emergency Response Unit. Air, mounted and marine unit sections of the Metropolitan Police are not overlooked, nor are their unique red-coloured Diplomatic Protection Group units and white-coloured Special Escort Group motorcycles escorting and protecting the most important of people.

# Discretion

No unpleasant or distressing images are featured; the right to privacy of victims, patients, witnesses is totally respected and observed as, of course, is the Terrorism Act 2000 in respect of national security. Hence, unmarked police vehicles and plain clothes police do not knowingly appear. No information other than that readily available by casually observing vehicle movement on the streets of the capital or by minimal research on websites and social media for information already in the public domain appears in these pages. The emphasis is very much to provide the reader with a pictorial record of vehicles to be seen by simply strolling through the streets of London.

# Geographical Scope

A single book could not cover the variety of different vehicles in use by the myriad of departments within the organisations covered in these pages. Instead, this book provides an overview, concentrating primarily on central London. Images taken in Camden, the City, Lambeth, Paddington and Whitechapel complement those captured in Soho and Whitehall.

# A Tribute

In presenting a publication of this nature, tribute is paid from the outset to the men and women of all the emergency services and to the clinical and medical staff receiving patients from many of those incidents. An unparalleled number of mass casualty major incidents occurred in London in the space of three months in 2017. These involved all the emergency services. Casualty figures are subject to change as this book went to press.

They were at Westminster Bridge (22 March: 5 killed, 50 injured plus the terrorist shot dead); London Bridge/Borough Market (3 June: 8 killed, 48 injured plus the three terrorists shot dead); the 24-storey-high, 129-flats, Grenfell Tower fire (14 June: 80 killed or missing presumed dead, 17 injured and still in hospital a week later), and Whadcoat Street/Seven Sisters Road, Finsbury Park (19 June: 1 dead, 9 injured, with the assailant arrested alive), not forgetting Manchester (22 May: 23 killed and 250 injured, with the killer blowing himself up).

Emergency service work is unpredictable and sometimes dangerous, dealing with a public often exposed to danger and violence, or suffering emotionally and physically from pain, loss, sorrow and anxiety. The care, compassion and concern of members of the emergency services – whether control room staff taking the initial calls, front line member of all the 999 services attending the scene, casualty bureau staff, disaster victim identification personnel, London Fire Brigade Urban Search teams or police family liaison officers – should never be overlooked. Nor should the violence and insult members of the 999 fraternity have to suffer on a daily basis when all they are doing is trying to help those in distress. Without the efforts of the highly trained emergency services personnel, ours would not be the civilised society that we all seek to enjoy and benefit from.

## Author's Note

Other than pre-arranged visits to London's Air Ambulance, Euston fire station, British Transport Police, Camden and attending the 2016 public open day at Paddington fire station, all images in this book were taken live from public areas of central London. All are dated between 2012 and 2017. Where night photography appears, to avoid distraction to drivers flash was not used in any photographs, all of which were taken in hand-held mode rather than using a tripod, owing to the suddenness with which vehicles would appear. Nothing has been added or removed from any image by electronic or any other means. Every effort has been taken to avoid featuring the readily identifiable faces of emergency service personnel. Where such images do occur it is with the permission of the individuals involved. Other than where indicated, all images were taken by the author.

# CHAPTER 1

# Ambulance

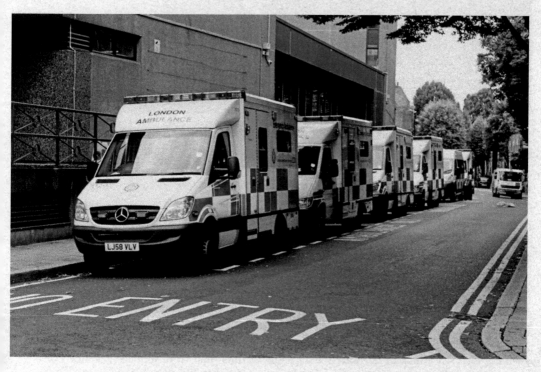

Emergency ambulances lined up at the side of the London Ambulance Service NHS Trust headquarters building.

## Introduction

Garrett Emmerson succeeded Dr Fionna Moore MBE as CEO of the London Ambulance Service NHS Trust (LAS) at the end of May 2017 – Andrew Grimshaw having been interim post holder for the intervening five months. The service has a staff of over 5,000 personnel working from seventy ambulance stations across the capital. Located on Waterloo Road,

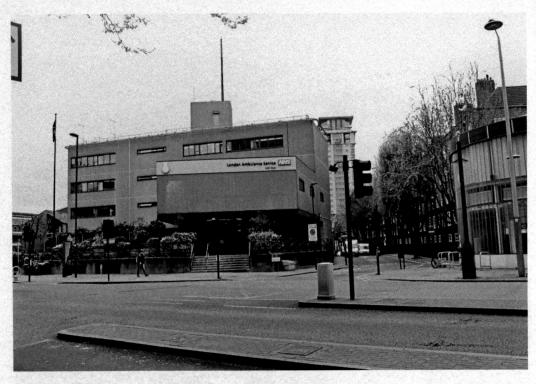

The front of London Ambulance Service Headquarters, Waterloo Road.

the distinctive LAS building serves not only as the headquarters complex complete with control room, but has an operational ambulance station at the rear in Frazier Street.

Many of London's hospitals are famous nationally and internationally, their size and diversity seeing a wide range of ambulance movements throughout the capital carrying patients for both emergency and elective surgery.

Facing the Palace of Westminster from the opposite embankment is St Thomas' Hospital. To one side of it lies the Florence Nightingale Museum and on the other side is the Evelina London Children's Hospital, the second largest children's provider in the capital. St Thomas' Hospital is central London's nearest hospital, complete with Accident & Emergency facilities. Its front entrance faces onto Westminster Bridge – scene of the mass casualty terrorist attack of 22 March 2017. Four victims died from injuries sustained on the bridge itself after having been run down by the terrorist's vehicle, which deliberately mounted the pavement before careering towards the Palace of Westminster. London Ambulance Service declared a Major Incident, resulting in a massive response from them. They were joined by hospital staff who rushed to the aid of around forty casualties strewn over a distance some 250 metres across the pavement and roadway of the bridge. The car hurtled on, crashing into the outer wall of the House of Commons in Bridge Street (a short continuation of Westminster Bridge), with the solitary assailant then running the few yards to the entrance just around the corner on Parliament Square.

Just inside the grounds of Parliament itself, unarmed Parliamentary and Diplomatic Protection Command's PC Keith Palmer bravely tried to stop the individual, who was

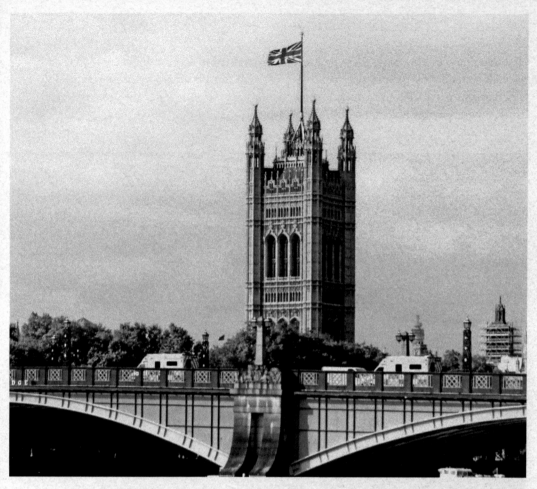

Two London emergency ambulances cross Lambeth Bridge, the Union Jack proudly billowing from the Palace of Westminster.

brandishing two knives according to eye witnesses. Tragically, PC Palmer made the ultimate sacrifice and succumbed to his injuries from the assailant's knife attack. A colleague shot the perpetrator dead before anyone else fell victim.

London's Air Ambulance (LAA) landed on Parliament Square with an Advanced Trauma Team and members of HART (the Hazardous Area Response Team) were equally quick to reach the scene.

London Ambulance Service, LAA, the police, fire brigade, RNLI, doctors and nursing staff spread across various London hospitals including St Thomas' Hospital and King's College Hospital – the latter a major trauma centre receiving the most critically injured seven victims – did a magnificent job in the most harrowing and difficult of circumstances. So too did many members of the public dashing to the aid of the victims on Westminster Bridge, as well as Foreign Office minister Tobias Ellwood – Conservative MP for Bournemouth East and now a member of the Privy Council – in trying to help PC Palmer as he lay stricken in New Palace Yard within the Palace of Westminster.

## Advanced Paramedic Practioners

First appointed in May 2014, these paramedics are trained to an even higher standard and normally attend only the most serious 1 to 2 per cent of calls where their life-saving skill is paramount. Their advanced qualification enables them to administer the more powerful drugs, otherwise only able to be given by a doctor.

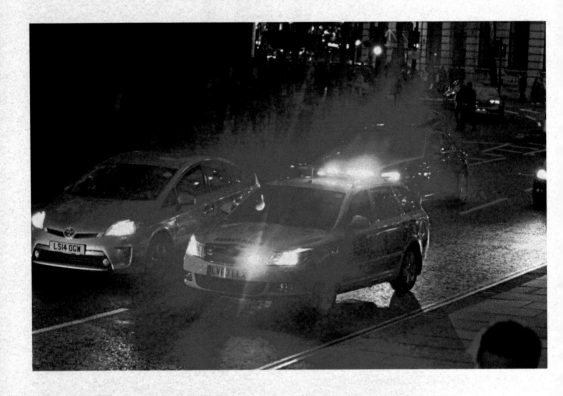

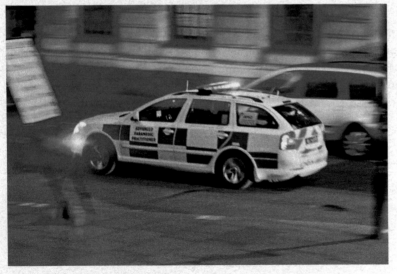

*Above*: An Advanced Paramedic Practioner believed to be attending a life-threatening road traffic collision on Waterloo Bridge.

*Left*: Dependant on traffic conditions, attendance at the incident is likely to be within two minutes.

# London's Air Ambulance

The crew of London's two air ambulances are funded by the NHS. The actual aircraft and leased land vehicles are funded by charitable donations. The newly appointed Chief Executive as of 19 April 2017 is Jonathan Jenkins and the Medical Director is Dr Gareth Davies – an Accident & Emergency and pre-hospital Care Consultant working at the Royal London. The helicopter is crewed by an advanced trauma doctor, an advanced trauma paramedic, and two pilots. They treated 1,864 patients in 2016 – 606 being road traffic victims, 500 as a result of stabbings or shootings, and 417 falls from height.

The original SA 365N Dauphin air ambulance was registered G-HEMS (Helicopter Emergency Medical Service) but its successor in 2000 had to be registered G-EHMS as identically formatted registration letters cannot be carried forward to subsequent aircraft. However, air ambulances up and down the country are commonly referred to as HEMS.

A donation of £2 million towards the cost of the £4 million purchase price of London's second MD902 Explorer air ambulance, registration G-LNDN, which went live in late January 2016, was made by London Freemasons – a magnificent gesture on their part. The government contributed £1 million from fines imposed upon the banks with the remaining £1 million being generously given by the public. Having two helicopters ensures one is always available if the other is away for service or repairs.

The distinctly marked fleet of four Skoda Octavia vJS estate cars and one Octavia Superb Outdoor estate (EJ 14 BWH) are due for replacement towards the end of the summer 2017. Of the present five vehicles, one car is designated for the Physician Response Unit, crewed by a doctor and Emergency Care Practitioner. They go to a patient's home, thereby helping prevent an unnecessary waste of ambulance resources. Two fully equipped cars are kept in immediate readiness if the helicopter is unable to fly (i.e. at night), is already committed, or the call is local. Except for the stretcher, both carry the identical equipment to that carried on the duty helicopter. The Advanced Trauma Team are mobilised 24/7 from the London Ambulance Service control room, where an air ambulance paramedic is on duty monitoring the incoming calls and deciding which ones can be best served by the air ambulance.

The current helipad, the highest air ambulance helipad in Europe, opened on 14 December 2011 is located 284 feet above ground level on top of the Royal London Hospital's seventeenth floor. A team of resident firefighters are present at each flight's arrival and take off, this being standard procedure for hospital rooftop helipads as there would be inevitable delay for the local fire brigade in gaining access.

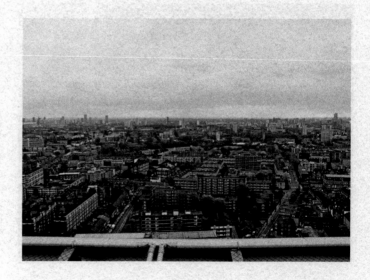

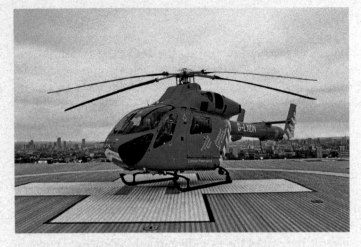

An immaculate G-LNDN in an immediate state of readiness for its next call. A dedicated high-speed lift enables arriving patients to be rapidly transferred to the Emergency Department at ground floor level.

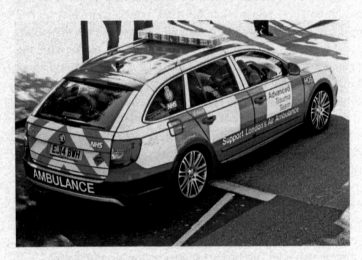

EJ14 BWH is London's Air Ambulance Skoda Superb Estate Outdoor version. (Image: Matt Holmes)

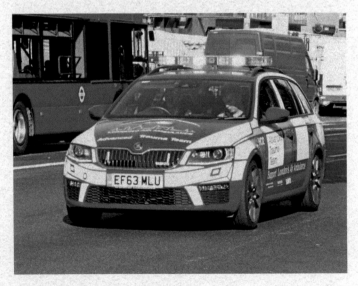

The Advanced Trauma Team consisting of a doctor and paramedic are also able to travel by road. EF63 MLU is one of four identical Skoda vRS models used for the purpose and is seen on an emergency response on 14 September 2016. (Image: Matt Holmes)

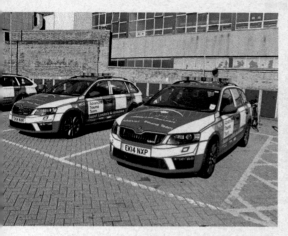 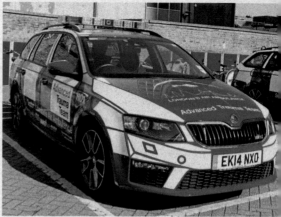

*Above left*: Identical vehicles are pictured in their designated bays at the Royal London Hospital, Whitechapel. Backup medical teams to a major incident can also be transported in these impressive looking Skoda Octavia vRS estate units.

*Above right*: The current batch of Skoda response vehicles bear an extremely smart livery well-suited to the body contour of the vehicles.

## Command Support Unit

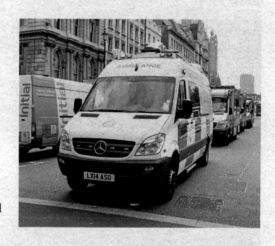

Equipped with green lights as well as blue, 2014's Command Support Unit is in direct contact with crews at the incident scene and with headquarters.

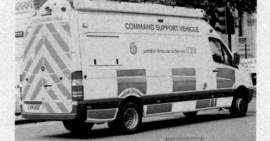

Strips of green flashing light at roof level are evident in this side view.

# Cycle Response Team

With its many alleyways and pedestrian precincts, the tightly compacted area of central London is ideal territory to be covered by the Cycle Response Team. Likewise, Heathrow Airport's terminals, Kingston town centre, and other congested areas of London such as the City of London and the St Pancras area, are covered by riders. They use lightweight but specially strengthened custom-built Rockhopper mountain bikes, with full medical kits including a defibrillator carried in the panniers for cardiac arrest patients. London Ambulance Service's Cycle Response Team (CRT) attends approximately 16,000 incidents a year and is able to resolve approximately 50 per cent of incidents on scene. Average response time to be in attendance at an incident is six minutes.

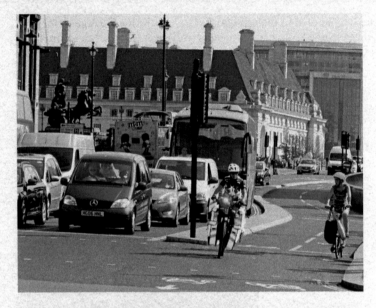

Fitted with siren and blue lights front and rear, congestion and red traffic lights are little obstacle when on an emergency.

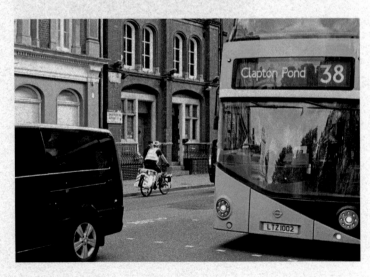

The versatility of a pedal cycle enables this paramedic rider, seen passing Theatreland's Shaftesbury Avenue street sign and shortly to turn left by Soho fire station, to access the lanes and pedestrianised areas of Chinatown without difficulty or delay. As can be seen, not all London buses are red!

# Driver Training Vehicles

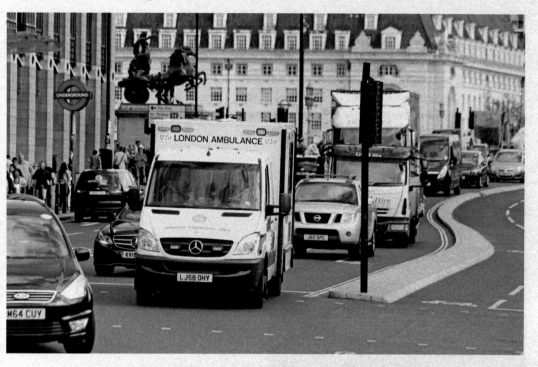

Now converted to a driver training vehicle, LJ58 OHY approaches Parliament Square.

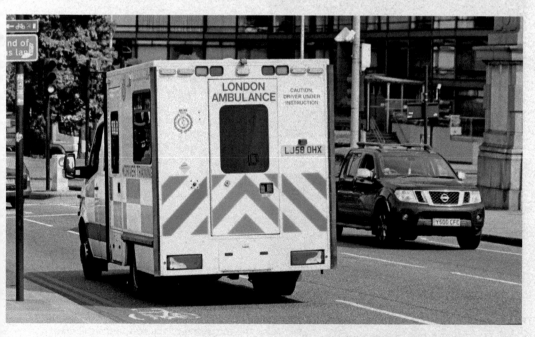

Sister driver training vehicle LJ58 OHX is about to negotiate Lambeth Road roundabout having crossed Lambeth Bridge.

## Emergency Ambulances

The Mercedes Sprinter-based chassis appeared on London's streets by 2005 and have remained the basis of the emergency response front line fleet ever since. It is no exaggeration to say that these days the ambulance service in general throughout the country is stretched to the hilt. Combine this with the adverse effect caused to so many people by alcohol and drugs, road traffic collisions, and assaults (sadly sometimes disgracefully committed against ambulance personnel only doing their best to help the patient), and it is no wonder crews and control staff have little time for rest and meal breaks during their arduous, emotional, and traumatic shifts.

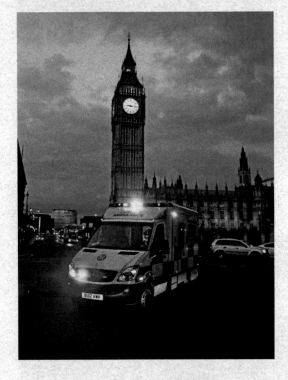

Mid-evening as a London ambulance on a shout heads for Whitehall, the Elizabeth Tower housing Big Ben – otherwise known as The Great Bell – the iconic backdrop.

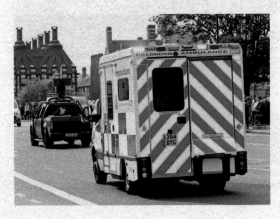

On 7 July 2016, Mercedes Sprinter ambulance LX64 DYG moved forward on the blues as the camera rolled as part of the recording of the brilliant three-part television series *Ambulance*, first shown by the BBC on 27 September 2016.

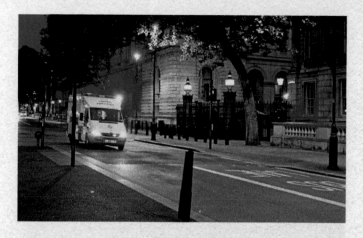

Whitehall is eerily quiet, devoid of tourists and traffic as the evening wears on. An ambulance passing the entrance to 10 Downing Street has no need to activate its sirens on this occasion.

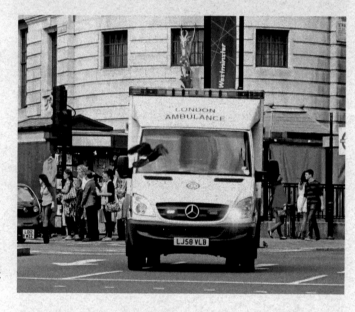

The driver, trained to both very high medical and driving standards, can be prepared for other road users creating hazards. Anticipating the hazardous movement of pigeons is not so easy!

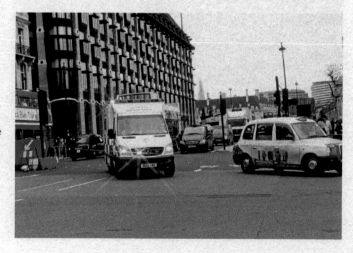

Yet another ambulance on a shout enters Parliament Square. Along with frequent responses from the other emergency services, it is hardly surprising many media broadcasts from central London are accompanied by the background of emergency vehicle sirens.

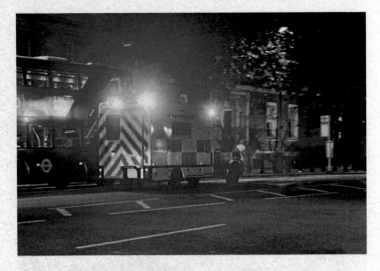

Blues vividly striking the side of the bus, an ambulance heads down Whitehall.

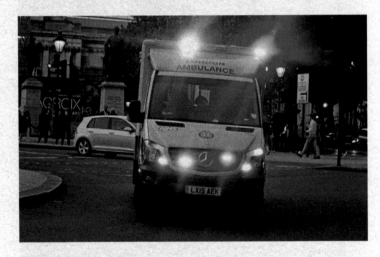

As dusk descends, an emergency ambulance leans into the bend at the bottom of Trafalgar Square.

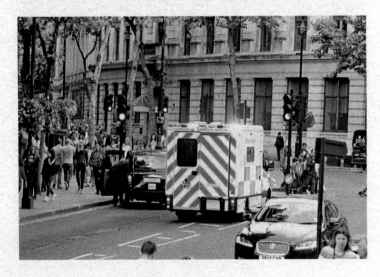

A taxi with its rear end sticking out is not the most helpful situation for the driver of the ambulance, now having to slow to negotiate what has unnecessarily become an awkward gap.

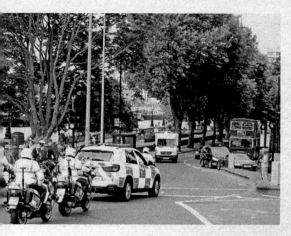
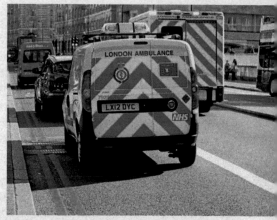

*Above left*: With their 999 colleagues wrong side of the road on a shout, a bevy of police vehicles come to a halt to enable the emergency ambulance to make progress. (Image: Margaret Boulter)

*Above right*: A Fiat van with large roof light bar being overtaken in York Road by a London ambulance on an emergency.

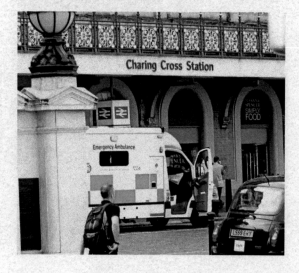

A variation on the familiar Mercedes chassis is this Fiat version in London Ambulance Service markings.

A very hot day in the capital with the driver's door open for a breath of fresh air sees the crew member snatching a quick glance of the newspaper before the next shout. Long may such moments be witnessed as our ambulance staff, whether in the control room or on the road, are so hard-pressed that the opportunity for a well-earned few moment's break is extremely rare.

# Hazardous Area Response Teams

HART is a 2009 NHS initiative providing specially trained medical personnel to tend patients in, as the name suggests, hazardous situations such as those involving chemicals, collapsed buildings, firearms or explosives, height, off-road, in water, and underground confined spaces such as entrapment under trains, to name just some. Their specialised equipment includes breathing apparatus, cutting equipment, rafts, and a Polaris off-road vehicle. Their skills were much in evidence at London's major incidents during the first half of 2017.

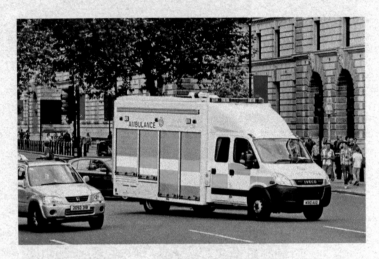

A HART vehicle crosses Parliament Square at routine speed.

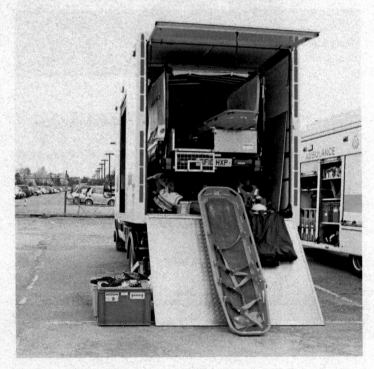

The rear box section is a roll on/roll off design, and once hydraulically lowered to the ground, the all-terrain Polaris unit is simply reversed out.

# Joint Response Teams

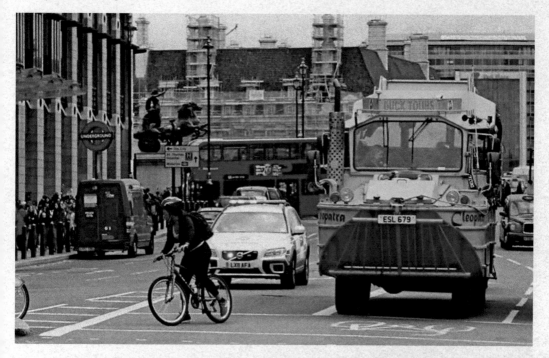

Other than for Red 1 emergency calls (cardiac or respiratory arrest), wherever they may occur, these vehicles are dedicated to respond to police calls in certain London boroughs on Thursday to Saturday evenings and nights, where their paramedic crew's medical skills are likely to be required.

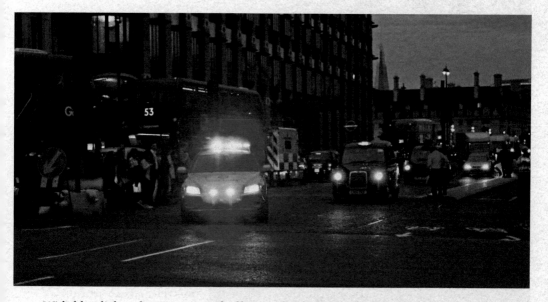

With blue lights showing to good effect in the darkness, this Volvo Joint Response Unit is making good progress, traffic having already moved over to assist its passage.

# Motorcycle Response Unit

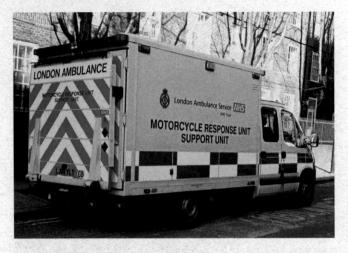

London Ambulance Service's crew cab Motorcycle Response Unit Support Unit parked near headquarters.

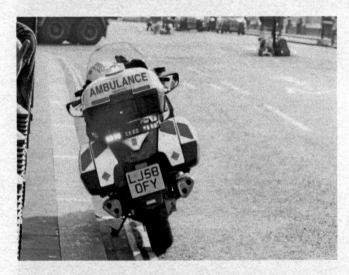

The motorcycle's paramedic rider is only a few metres away, tending a patient inside the entrance to Westminster Underground station.

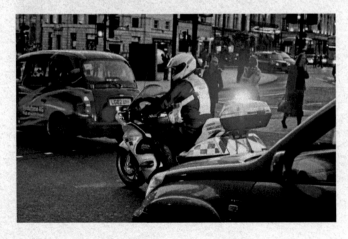

With the penetrating sound of the machine's siren bouncing off the buildings, this rider adeptly weaves through Trafalgar Square's evening traffic.

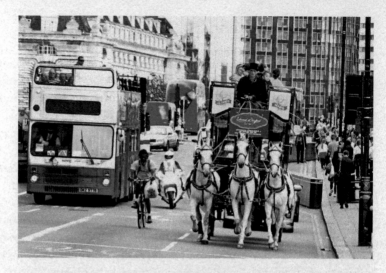

The horses pulling the replica bus remain perfectly disciplined despite the rapidly approaching motorcycle response unit on an emergency call, its siren now silenced as it approaches them.

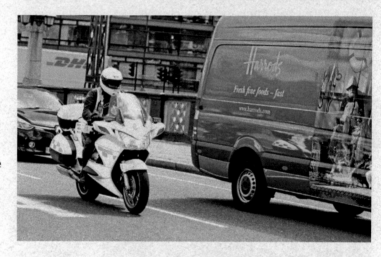

The motorcycle response unit is seen here passing a Harrods van. The store is world famous for quality, as is the care administered by the London Ambulance Service.

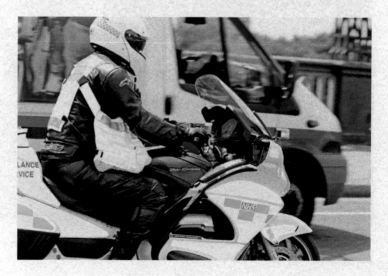

A van gives the motorcyclist on the blues crossing Lambeth Bridge room to safely pass.

# Rapid Response Vehicles (RRV)

In addition to Advanced Paramedic Practioners, Advanced Trauma Team and Joint Response Unit vehicles already featured, this section focuses upon cars, estates and 4x4s simply marked 'Ambulance'. They are placed under the generic heading 'Rapid Response Vehicles'. All are in experienced, medically trained hands, whether the individual's role is duty officer, first response, incident officer, incident response officer, paramedic, paramedic team leader, scene commander, or senior officer, to name but a few.

It is a misconception that siren blasting and blues lights pulsating clears roadways for the emergency service vehicle. Any 999 driver will tell you the truth is it does not! Emergency service drivers have to be extremely careful, especially travelling on the wrong side of the road and/or at high speed as motorists, cyclists and pedestrians often have little time to react to their approach. The problem is compounded if the member of the public is very young or elderly, physically or mentally infirm, deaf or partly sighted, under the influence of drugs or alcohol, listening through headphones or on their mobile phone. Sadly a very small minority of people choose to be deliberately obstructive towards the approach of an emergency vehicle. Thus, the utmost vigilance on the part of the highly trained emergency service vehicle driver is demanded at all times.

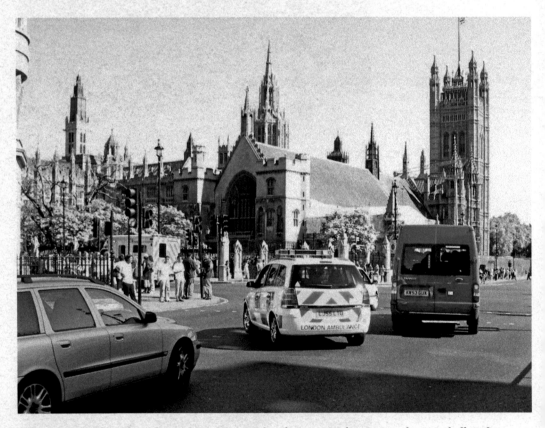

The ambulance has cleared a path and is now heading up Bridge Street, the Vauxhall Zafira paramedic estate not far behind.

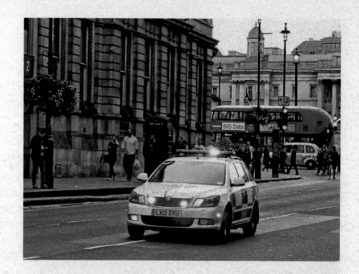

Accelerating hard, the paramedic at the wheel of a Skoda RRV enjoys the rarity of a clear stretch of road at the top of Whitehall.

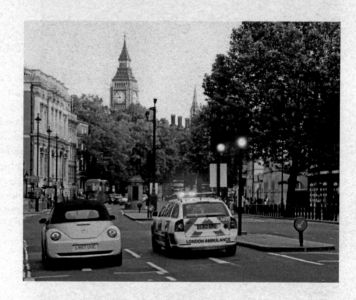

Relatively clear conditions for Whitehall remain as this Skoda RRV, shortly to pass Banqueting House, heads towards London's world-famous Big Ben.

Hopefully the tourist sat on the bollard near the RRV on Horse Guards Parade will shortly move as all these are remotely controlled and at the press of a button retract out of sight. If that happens he might need the paramedic's services!

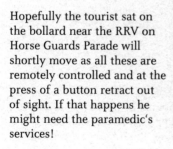

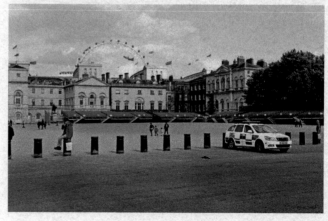

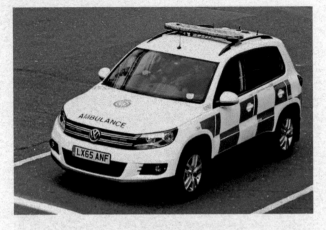

Replacing the older rapid response fleet are VW Tiquan saloons, one of the earlier models to join the London Ambulance Service fleet pictured here.

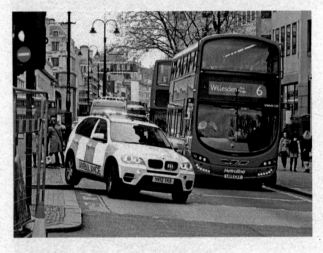

Due to roadworks blocking the entrance to Strand, a short stretch of the eastbound dual carriageway behind the fencing is clear of vehicular traffic. The paramedic team leader's vehicle is able to take advantage and very gently negotiate the central reservation to regain the correct side of the road, thereby avoiding the westbound congestion.

## NHS Blood & Transplant

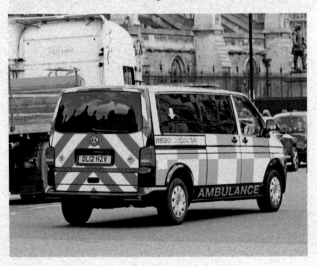

A VW used to transport a National Organ Retrieval Service team from its regional base passes the Palace of Westminster.

# British Red Cross Society

Invaluable support to Londoners is given by the British Red Cross Society. Exactly the same is to be said in respect of St John Ambulance. Both organisations thrive on the active support of volunteer members who willingly and freely give their time to help others.

*Right*: One of three similar units operated by the British Red Cross in the capital, this Emergency Response Unit is providing support for a road run through central London.

*Below*: The road run has not yet started but already this British Red Cross ambulance crew are attending a medical emergency in Parliament Square.

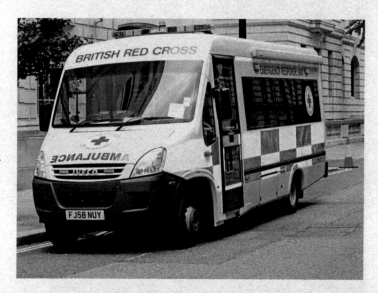

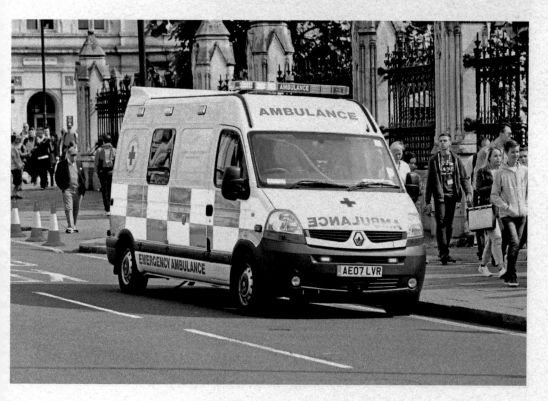

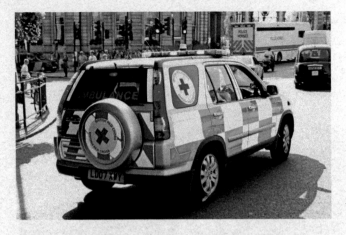

A Honda CR-V on the blues heading for the Pall Mall area.

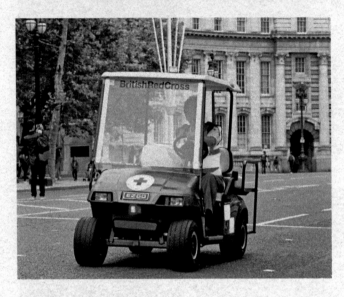

A versatile buggy equally able to traverse footpaths and parkland, plenty of which adjoin The Mall along which it was headed.

## St John Ambulance

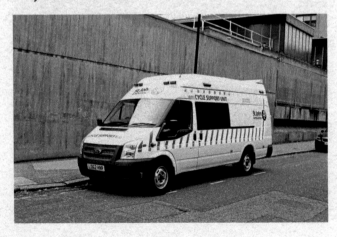

Parked adjacent to the London Ambulance Service Headquarters is St John Ambulance's Ford Transit Cycle Support Unit.

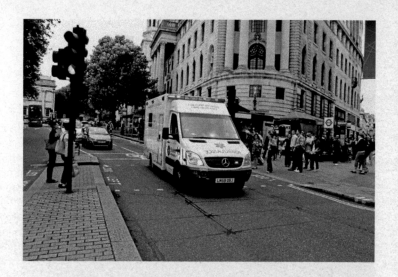

With siren reverberating off the high-sided South African embassy in Trafalgar Square, traffic froze to allow this children's ambulance unobstructed passage down the inside lane.

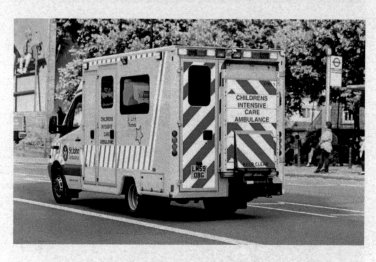

These dedicated St John ambulances are a frequent sight in central London. Evelina London Children's Hospital is located adjacent to St Thomas' Hospital.

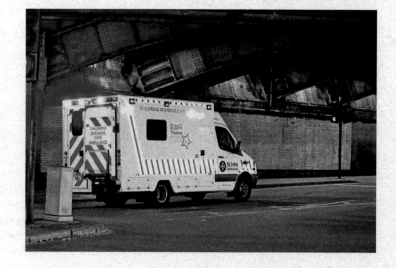

Although it was broad daylight, this children's ambulance was photographed in the semi-darkness of Westminster Bridge Road as it raced outbound under the arches carrying the railway tracks above into the platforms of Waterloo station.

# Private Firms

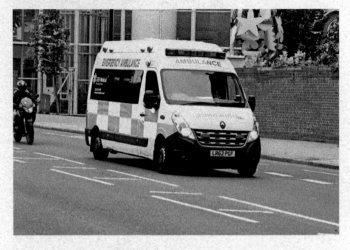

Numerous private firms with modern ambulances are a frequent sight in central London. Space limitations unfortunately mean only a very small number of random images can be shown in this volume. A Renault ambulance of ERS Medical passes the Evelina London Children's Hospital.

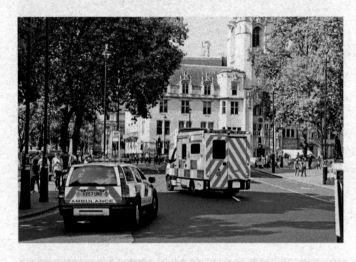

Non-NHS Volvo estate of Docklands Medical Services halts to allow a London Ambulance Service vehicle on a shout to pass. In the background of this Parliament Square image is the Supreme Court.

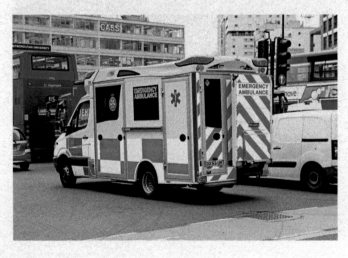

The distinctive roof line of a UK Specialist Ambulance Service Mercedes ambulance is evident in this shot as it makes its way outbound on the A11 from the City of London.

# CHAPTER 2

# Fire & Rescue

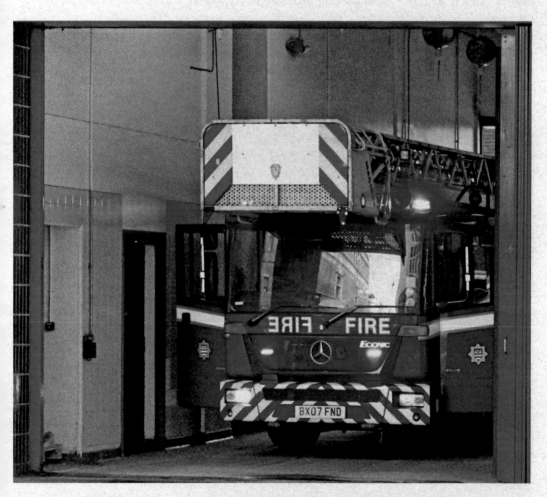

Soho's turntable ladder having reversed into its bay. (Image: Margaret Boulter)

# Introduction

From 1937 until 2007, the brigade's headquarters was located on Albert Embankment, near Lambeth Bridge. It is now located at 169 Union Street, London SE1 0LL. A pop-up brigade museum opened on 9 November 2016 in Lambeth High Street at the back of the old headquarters.

The London Fire and Emergency Planning Authority run the brigade, which is under the command of the inspirational Dany Cotton, QFSM, who was promoted following the retirement of Ron Dobson CBE, QFSM, FIFireE on 31 December 2016. Dany is the first female officer to command the brigade, which is one of the world's largest with almost 6,000 personnel, of which 5,096 are operational firefighters. It is the only brigade in the country where all of its firefighters are full time as opposed to a mixture of full- and part-time firefighters.

Despite a rise in population in figures announced by the brigade in early June 2016, fire calls in London are down 23.18 per cent over the past five years – a remarkable tribute to the brigade's proactive educational policy, smoke alarms and sprinklers in helping reduce fires, the general public happy to take advantage of and heed the free and willingly given professional fire safety advice. Many of the brigade's pumping appliances carry fire safety advice in large lettering, a vital and distinctive source of educating the public and very much part of their successful efforts to make London a safer place.

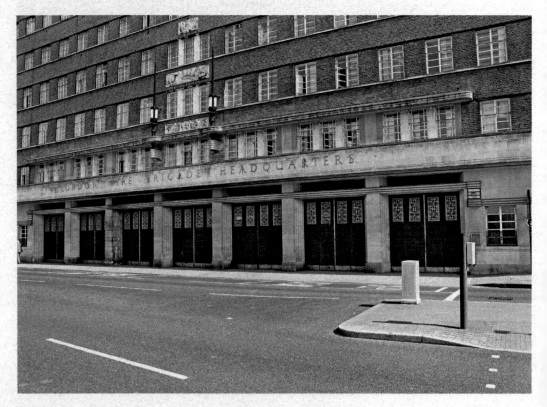

The wording 'London Fire Brigade Headquarters' can still be seen above Lambeth fire station's seven appliance bay doors.

# Aerial Appliances

For many years London's aerial appliances were automatically mobilised to a vast array of incidents. That is no longer the case, an aerial appliance now only attending when specifically requested or as part of the pre-determined attendance to higher risk premises. Only becoming aware from Twitter of the closing stages of a six-pump incident in Gerrard Place, Soho, on 10 July 2016 a range of appliance movements were nevertheless able to be recorded. This included two turntable ladders.

---

### Appliances with their registrations, call sign and home station seen at or in standby mode adjacent to the Gerrard Place, Soho incident

PUMPS

| | | |
|---|---|---|
| RY52 BKA | A322 | A32 Hornsey |
| EU03 DHM | A242 | A24 Soho |
| RL03 LVX | H222 | H22 Lambeth |
| AE56 SFZ | G271 | G27 North Kensington |
| AE57 FNO | A281 | A28 Dowgate |
| AE57 FNR | A211 | A21 Paddington |
| AE07 HWF | A231 | A23 Euston |
| AE07 HWP | G341 | G34 Chelsea |
| AE07 HWR | A241 | A24 Soho |

TURNTABLE LADDERS

| | | |
|---|---|---|
| BX07 FND | A243 | A24 Soho |
| BX07 GUE | A213 | A21 Paddington |

COMMAND UNITS

| | | |
|---|---|---|
| WX56 VCE | CU2 | A30 Islington |
| WX07 NVG | CU8 | G35 Fulham |

FIRE INVESTIGATION UNIT

| | | |
|---|---|---|
| AE56 SFU | OK16 | A28 Dowgate |

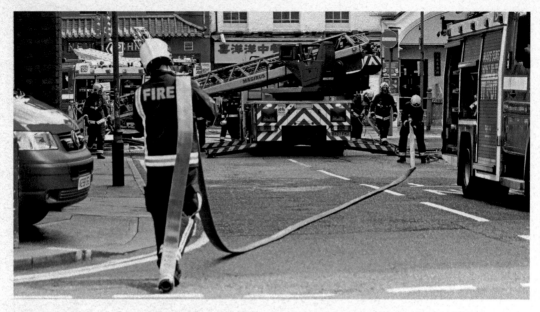

A hose is now being made up as the Soho aerial appliance makes ready to return to its home station.

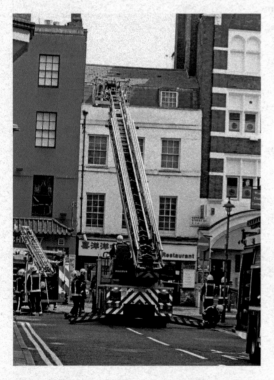
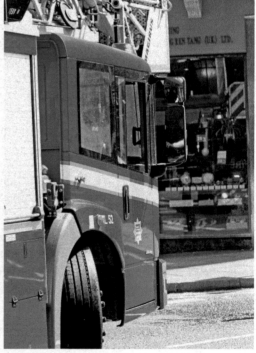

*Above left*: Soho's ladders are now being stowed before, uniquely, the aerial appliance makes a 100 metre journey in reverse on the blues back to its home station.

*Above right*: Gently reversing under the watchful eye of driver and a bank person, front blues reflecting in the corner shop window, the machine commences its 180 degree turn to enter its bay.

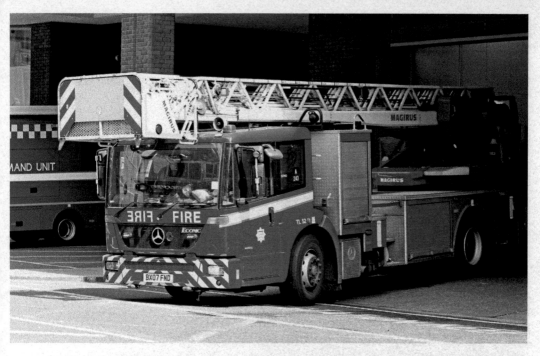

As Soho's turntable ladder almost completes reversing into its bay, North Kensington's pump ladder (on standby duty in the middle bay) prepares to mobilise on a shout. Blue light from the pump ladder is reflected in the base of the side locker behind the cab of the turntable ladder. (Image: Margaret Boulter)

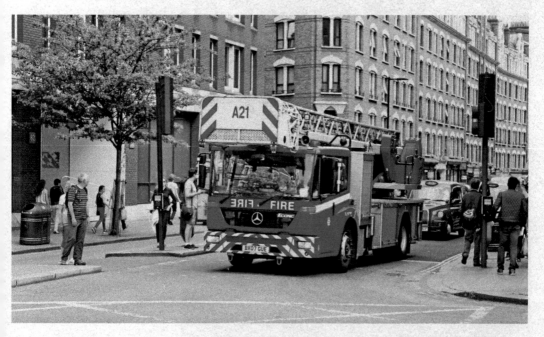

The Paddington aerial appliance, having been positioned in Gerrard Street at the Soho incident, heads back to station A21 via Cambridge Circus.

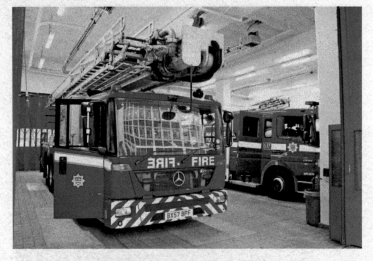

Reserve aerial ladder platform BX57 BPF is pictured deputising for Soho's regular turntable ladder away on planned maintenance.

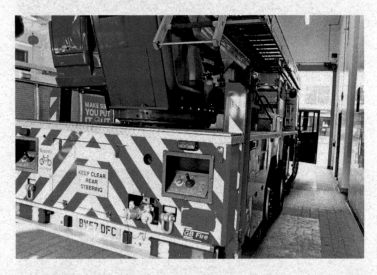

Yet again an aerial ladder platform was deputising, this time BV57 DFC. My thanks for permission to obtain the rear shot from within the fire station.

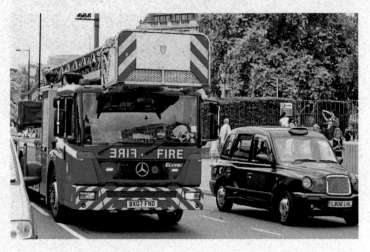

With siren blasting as it fights its way through heavy traffic, Soho's regular machine is pictured near the Tower of London. The grill-mounted poppy is a feature often to be seen on Soho's two regular pumps and turntable ladder.

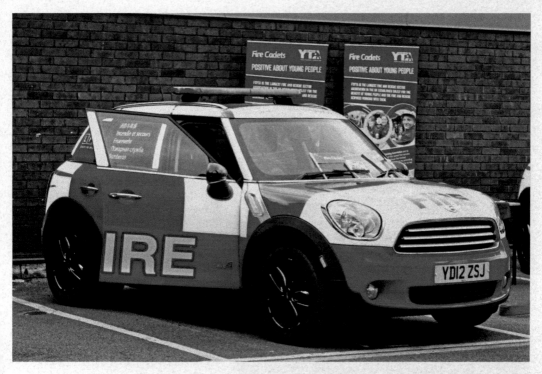

Introduced originally as small fire response units for the 2012 Olympic Games site in east London were five Mini Cooper Countryman saloons. This example, surrounded by literature for the excellent 'Positive About Young People' London Fire Brigade Cadets scheme, was on display at the Paddington fire station 2016 public open day.

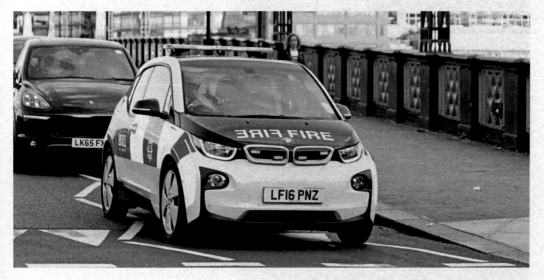

One of a batch of fifty-seven BMWi3 ultra low emission and hybrid electric cars delivered to the brigade from late 2016 onwards crosses Lambeth Bridge.

## Command Units

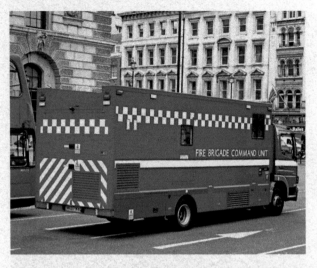

The brigade runs eight Command Units, enabling the largest of incidents to be sectorised with a command unit allocated to each if need be. The Fulham-based Command Unit is seen on a routine journey in central London.

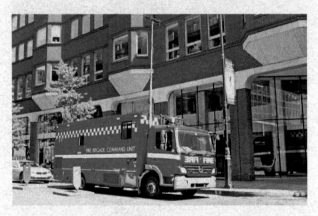

At the Soho restaurant fire previously mentioned, two command units were in attendance. Islington's Command Unit, mast erected, is pictured at work a few metres from the fire station in Shaftesbury Avenue, the incident just around the corner.

## Detection, Investigation and Monitoring (CBRN)

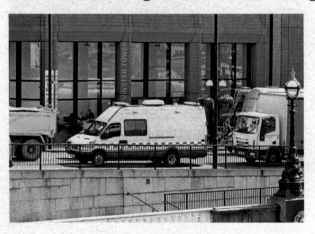

Helping keep Londoner's safe, this unit with specialist scientific crew is deployed to incidents where CBRN (Chemical, Biological, Radiological and Nuclear) materials may be involved. Similar units exist on a regional basis throughout the UK.

# Fireboats

The brigade's river fire station lies immediately opposite the Lambeth land-based fire station. London Fire Brigade has two identical 1999 Alnmaritec (Northumberland) built vessels, *Fire Dart* (No. 4768) and *Fire Flash* (No. 4769). One is kept operational and the other in reserve. *Fire Flash* (nearest camera) and *Fire Dart* are pictured moored at the River fire station in this early April 2017 image.

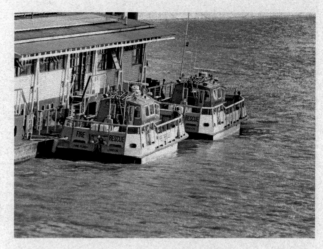

The duty fireboat attends incidents such as fires onboard vessels, fires in riverside property, and boat collision or sinking. It also acts in support of the RNLI and Metropolitan Police in rescuing people from the River Thames and may well be first in attendance at such incidents.

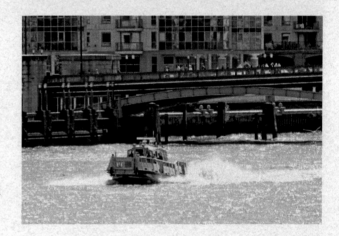

In celebration of Her Majesty becoming this country's longest reigning monarch at 63 years and 219 days, on 9 September 2015 a small pageant sailed up the river to the Palace of Westminster. The Royal Rowbarge *Gloriana* is facing the preserved London Fire Brigade Dunkirk veteran *Massey Shaw*, modern fireboat *Fire Dart*, and police launch MP1 *Patrick Colquhoun II*.

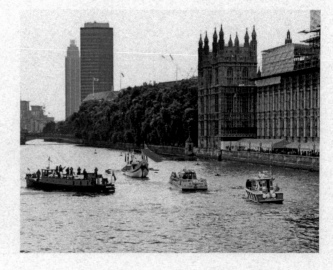

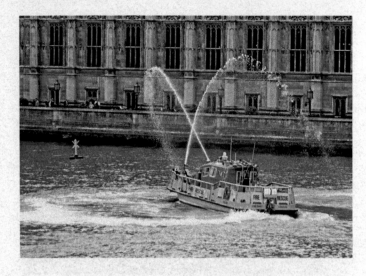

The sight of *Fire Dart,* jets crossed and spinning rapidly through 360 degrees, was a memorable one for the large crowd watching from Westminster Bridge.

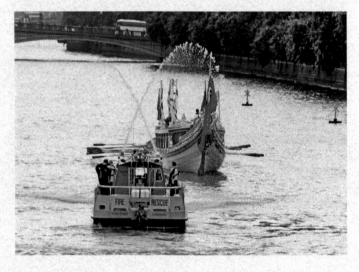

Continuing its tribute, *Fire Dart* then moved forward taking up position facing the royal rowbarge.

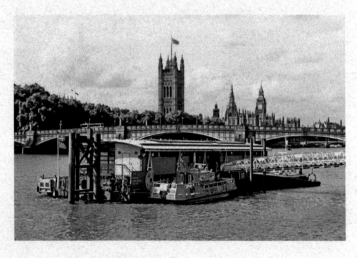

The magnificent backdrop to the London River fire station is the Palace of Westminster, pictured in this 2012 shot taken from Albert Embankment.

# Fire Investigation Units

Fire Investigation Vehicles are all stationed at fire investigation headquarters within Dowgate fire station, which is also the home to the brigade's arson response team and its three search dogs. Covering all of London the units attend fatal fires, suspicious fire-related incidents, those with an unknown cause, and incidents at which four or more crews are in attendance. This unit blasts through Tower Hill on the blues.

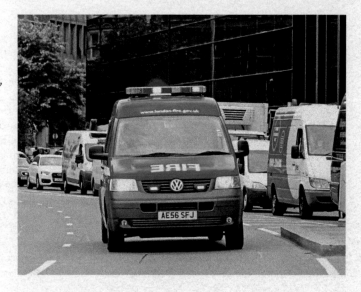

Mobile to an incident and badly hampered by the usual heavy traffic conditions in Strand, this Fire Investigation Unit eventually breaks free.

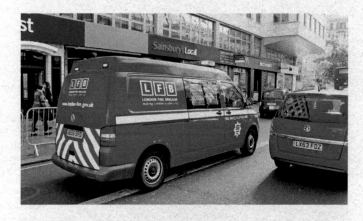

Parked on the pavement outside the pedestrian entrance to Soho fire station is Fire Investigation Unit Oscar Kilo One Six. The station's pump ladder is just visible to the right of the picture at the Chinatown incident.

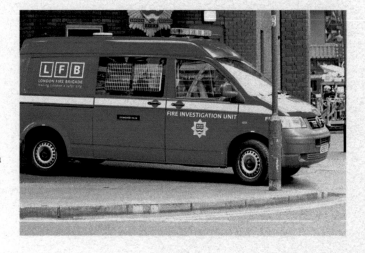

# Fire Rescue Units

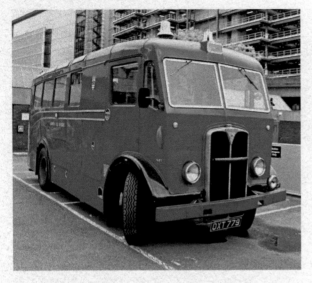

Pictured recently but long since retired, a beautifully restored AEC Regent/Merryweather Emergency Tender seen at the 2016 Paddington Open Day. This appliance went to the then station D61 Lambeth and thereafter to C21 Shoreditch before entering the reserve fleet in 1970s. All credit to Mike Cotton, a Watch Manager at Tottenham fire station, for his preservation efforts and the thoroughly deserved Brigade title of 'Volunteer of the Year 2016' for his unstinting efforts in respect of this and other preserved appliances. Very well done Mike!

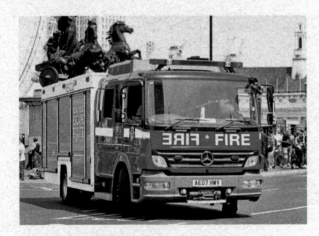

Paddington's Fire Rescue Unit is pictured emerging from Victoria Embankment. These vehicles carry a wide array of rescue equipment including portable generators and floodlighting along with heavy lifting gear, winch, cutting equipment, extended duration breathing apparatus and chemical protection.

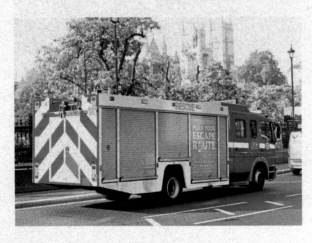

This reserve Fire Investigation Unit will shortly emerge from Bridge Street to pass Westminster Abbey, visible in the background.

# Operational Support Unit/Incident Response Unit

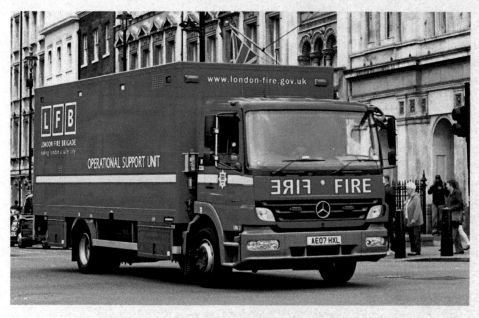

These vehicles carry large quantities of breathing apparatus or damage/salvage gear, as well as palletised loads of special equipment. An immaculately kept Wandsworth unit (OSU 2) exits Parliament Street.

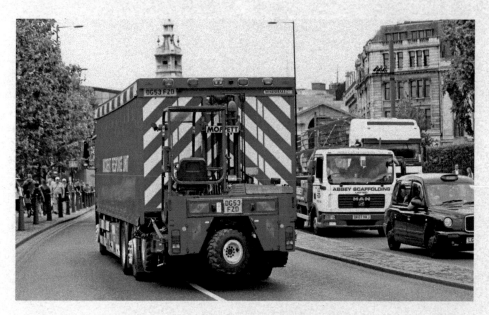

Another vehicle able to transport vital equipment to the fireground is the Incident Response Unit. Fitted with curtain sides and rear-mounted demountable fork lift truck is this M.A.N. vehicle, part of a 2003 government initiative to help equip brigades on a regional basis with an enhanced response to mass casualty incidents. This vehicle can carry gas-tight suits, inflatable tents, as well as casualty decontamination clothing and showers.

# Pumping Appliances

The workhorses of the brigade are fire engines, commonly referred to as fire appliances, capable of pumping water hence being known as pumps. Some carry subsidiary ladders while mainly acting as a pumping appliance while others perform that function but also carry a 13.5-metre-long triple extension ladder, hence the expression pump ladder. Due to the pumping appliance's versatility with its ladder carrying arrangements, an alternative title for the machine is Dual Purpose Ladder or DPL. The pumps on front line duty in London at the start of 2017 dated as far back as 2002/03. Fifty-three Mercedes/Emergency One (UK) Ltd pumping appliances are coming on stream during the year, nineteen delivered by mid-May 2017.

The area of central London this book features is covered principally by crews and appliances from Soho and Lambeth fire stations. However, appliances from other London fire stations can often be seen due to a number of other stations in the vicinity. Listed alphabetically under their home station is a selection of appliances from this variety of stations.

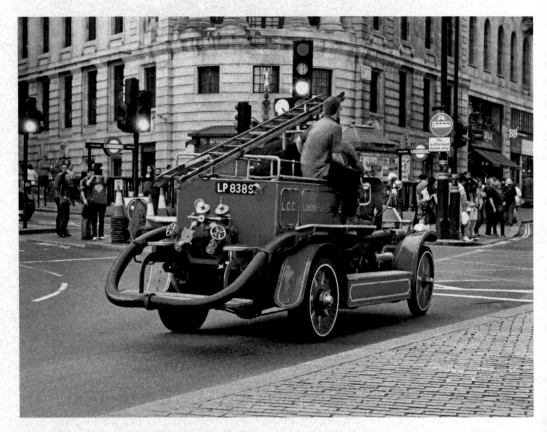

Now in the ownership of The Royal College of Science Motor Club, part of Imperial College, London, is early London Fire Brigade motorised appliance LP 8389, pictured on the evening of 9 July 2016 leaving Trafalgar Square. Delivered in April 1916 as No. 66 pump, it was stationed at the then Vauxhall fire station. Design and equipment has evolved somewhat over the century!

# Brixton

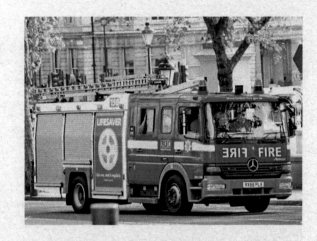

Brixton's 2005/06-registered pump heads up towards London's Theatreland. Appliances registered after these dates were fitted with full-width roof bar blue lights.

# Chelsea

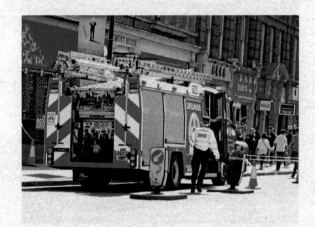

Chelsea's pump ladder about to depart from the Soho fireground on their next shout. With the crew having moved the cones blocking Shaftesbury Avenue, the policewoman on traffic duty kindly moves up to replace them after their departure.

# Dowgate

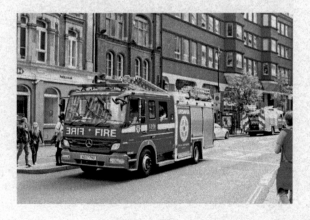

Now released from the six-pump fire in Gerrard Place, Dowgate's appliance heads for its home station. Paddington's pump ladder is in the background.

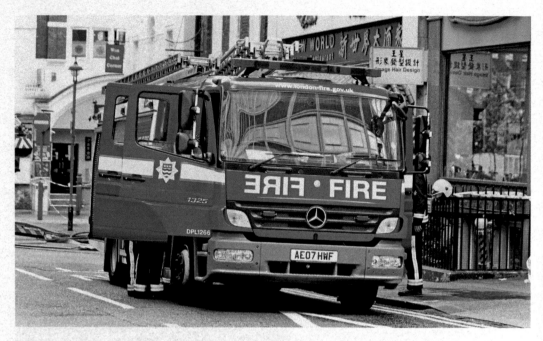

Euston's 2007-registered pump ladder still in immaculate condition, fitting testimony to the care and attention lavished on the appliance by various duty watches and brigade workshops. This appliance was replaced in early 2017.

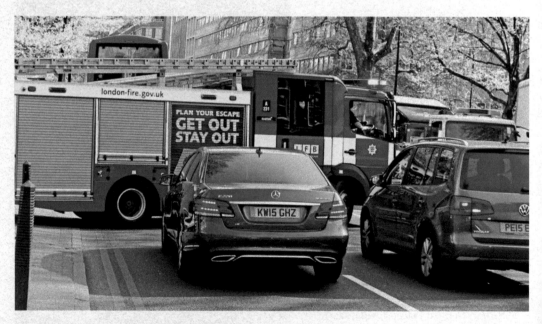

Turning out into dense traffic on 6 April 2017, station A23 Euston's new Mercedes/Emergency One pump ladder, registration WO66 HGG, fleet number DPL158, will then turn towards King's Cross.

As traffic in front crawls forward, the new pump now very slowly makes its way across the box junction on Euston Road as it nears its home station.

Both of Euston's appliances pictured on their home station. The new pump ladder and 2005-registered Fire Rescue Unit (RX05 AVD, FRU16) have the benefit of a raised roof level rear crew compartment.

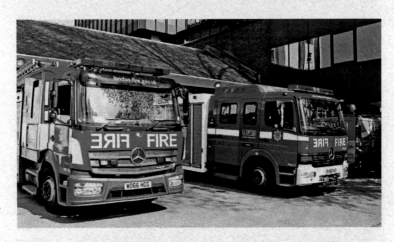

Tony Marshall, a justifiably proud Watch Manager, stood by the station's new appliance. The author's thanks are extended to Tony and both his crews at Euston for their friendly welcome and to firefighter Keiron Maden for kindly positioning the new appliance for the camera.

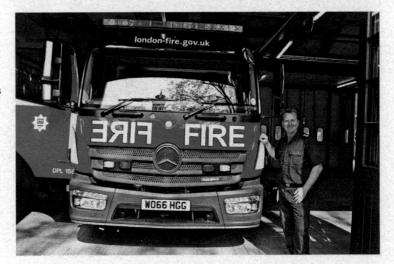

# Hornsey

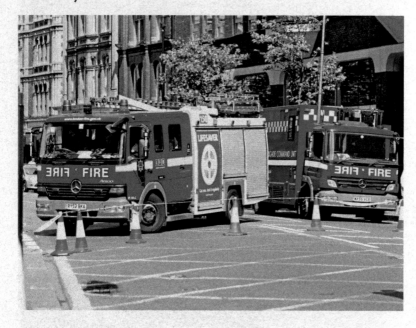

Hornsey are attending a shout elsewhere on Soho's ground and are obliged to seek an alternative route due to the continuing closure of Shaftesbury Avenue.

# Lambeth

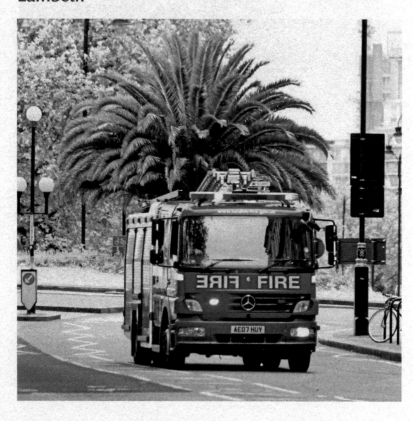

Millbank roundabout at its junction with Lambeth Bridge and Horseferry Road is the rather picturesque setting for the Lambeth appliance now accelerating hard towards Parliament Square.

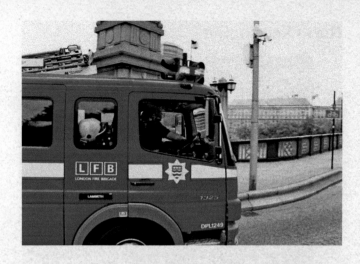

Storming up onto Lambeth Bridge from the Albert Embankment end, the Lambeth pump ladder follows a route it has no doubt taken hundreds of times in its twelve-year history.

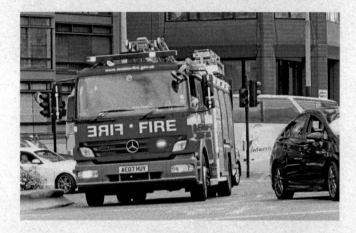

The camber on Lambeth Road roundabout evident in this image, this shout will take the appliance down Lambeth Road.

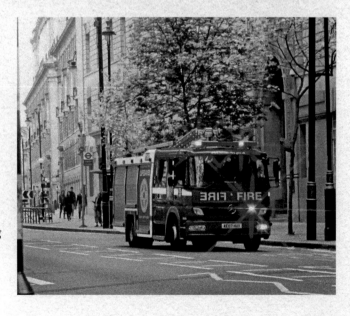

With a star-8 filter fitted to the camera lens, the resulting effect vividly captures the grill flasher on Lambeth's pump ladder as it heads towards Abingdon Street.

## North Kensington

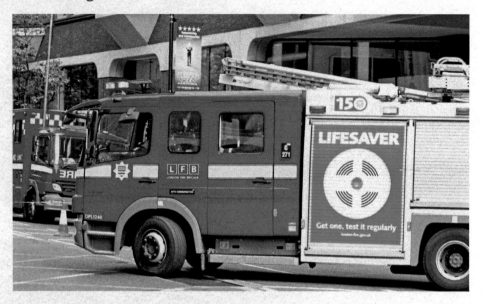

North Kensington, on standby in Soho fire station, are now mobile to a fresh call on Soho's fireground on the busy Sunday afternoon of 10 July 2016. Chelsea, Hornsey and Lambeth appliances have already been seen mobilising to separate incidents.

## Soho

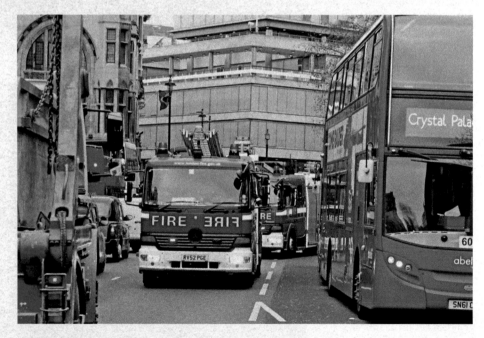

Soho's two pumps cross onto the opposing carriageway in Cockspur Street as oncoming traffic moves over, allowing them to pass the bus in safety.

EU03 DHM, running as a Soho pump, is pictured in attendance at a minor air conditioning unit incident involving a coach parked near London's South Bank. A small extension ladder has been shipped from the appliance's gantry to facilitate rooftop examination of the effected vehicle.

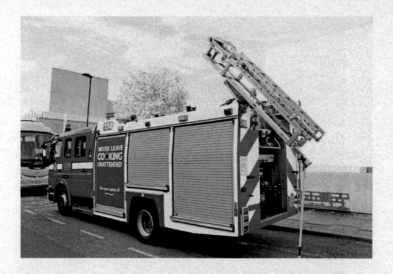

This time the appliance acting as Soho's pump (i.e. without a triple-extension ladder) heads down Whitehall passing a smart looking 'New Bus for London' in former London General livery.

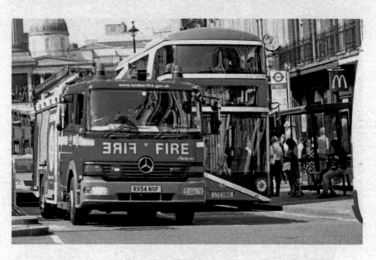

Returning appliances briefly block Shaftesbury Avenue, using their blue lights to warn traffic and pedestrians as they reverse into their respective bays. Mercedes Atego pump RX54 NXF is pictured on 5 April 2017 backing into its bay under the watchful eye of a crew member acting as banksperson.

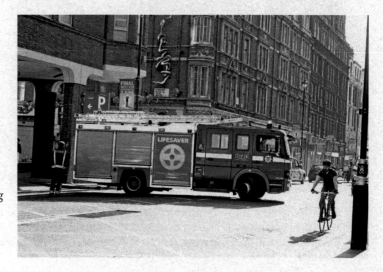

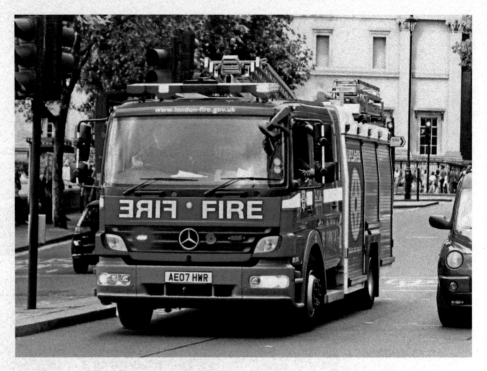

With traffic lights on green, Soho's immaculate pump ladder is able to accelerate through the normally congested junction with London's Strand.

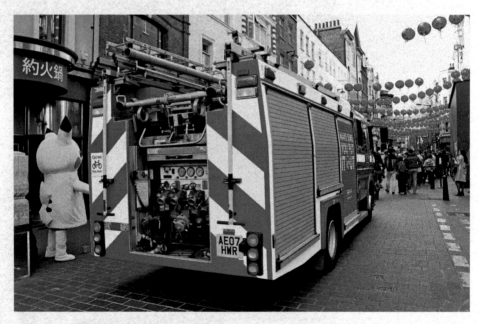

Soho firefighters are well respected and fully integrated into the community they serve. Here, the station's pump ladder is pictured edging through the heart of Soho's Chinatown district. A lookalike of leading character Pikachu from the Pokémon franchise watches intently!

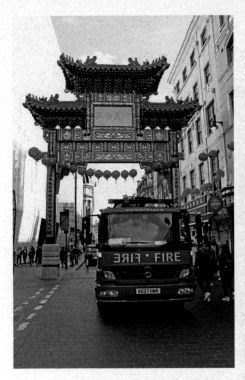
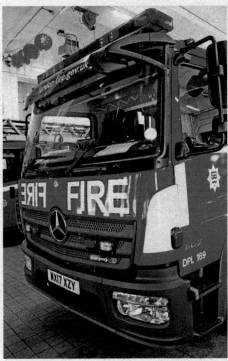

*Above left*: The final shot of AE07 HWR is of the appliance on its own station ground, the ornamental arch forming a truly beautiful backdrop.

*Above right*: Chinese lanterns seen in the previous two images can often be seen in Soho fire station's appliance room, a very visible indication of the goodwill and close association that exists between brigade personnel and the community they serve.

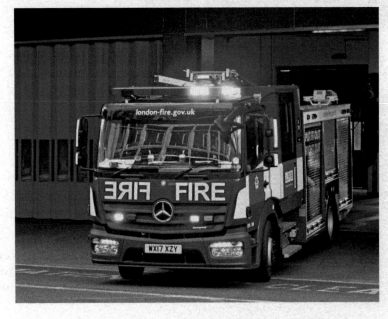

Captured reversing back into its bay on Sunday 14 May 2017 and only on the run for a few days is Soho's new pump ladder, the strength of its blue lights leaving no one in any doubt as to its presence! (Image: Matt Holmes)

## Southgate

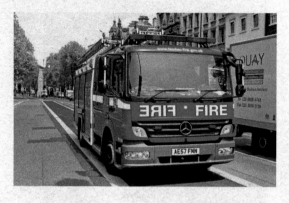

Paying a visit to central London is Southgate's pump ladder parked and unattended, with the crew 'off the run' while they familiarise themselves with nearby risks. The Cenotaph in Whitehall is visible in the background.

## Southwark

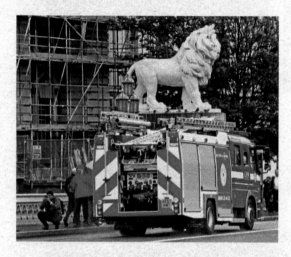

Dominated by the statue of the South Bank Lion, the former Southwark-based fire station appliance AE07 HWT is pictured having just crossed Westminster Bridge. The station closed in January 2015.

## Royal Household (Buckingham Palace) Fire Service Vehicle

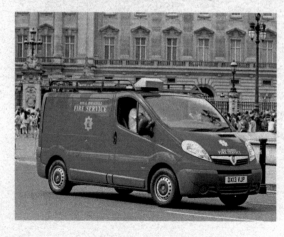

The Royal Household have their own vehicle kept within its grounds, which can occasionally seen on the adjoining public roads. Sightings of earlier vehicles of the same size and appearance suggest its prime role is salvage, the most priceless of artefacts being within the Palace.

# National Firefighters Memorial

The National Memorial to fallen firefighters in Sermon Lane lies in the shadow of St Paul's Cathedral. Annually, on the second Sunday in September, a memorial service is held. Wreaths from families, all the fire and rescue services in the country, pensioner's associations, and from other emergency services and organisations are laid in remembrance of those who gave their lives in the Second World War and subsequently in peacetime.

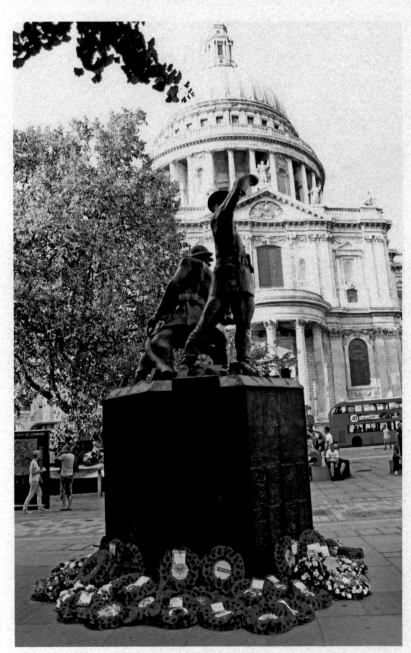

Such poignancy in the family tributes following 2016's wreath laying, it would be difficult not to have a profound effect on all who were to read them.

# CHAPTER 3

# Police

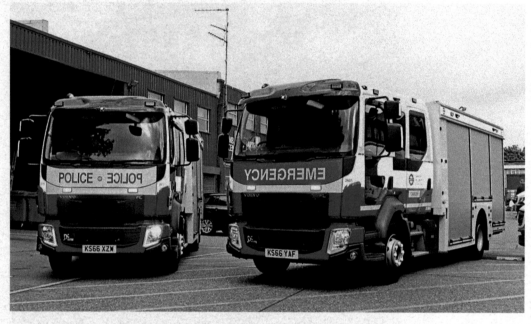

British Transport Police, Transport for London and London Underground working in total harmony.

## The Metropolitan Police Service – New Scotland Yard

Approximately 32,000 police officers, 9,000 non-police support staff, over 1,600 Police Community Support Officers and around 3,200 members of the special constabulary form the Metropolitan Police in early 2017. Upon his retirement after five years in command, Sir Bernard Hogan-Howe was replaced as Commissioner by Cressida Dick, who took command from Acting Commissioner Craig Mackay on 10 April 2017 as the first female Commissioner of the force.

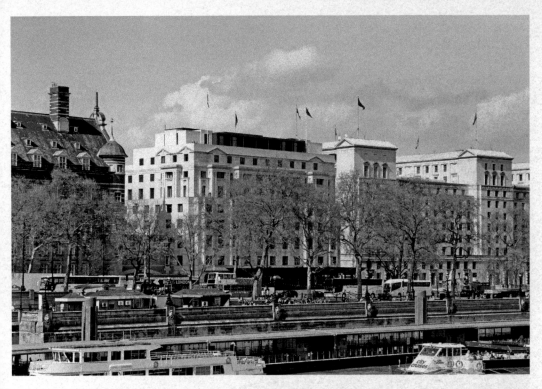

The Metropolitan Police Service HQ on Victoria Embankment viewed from Westminster Bridge. The HQ is located opposite the South Bank's London Eye.

## Air Support

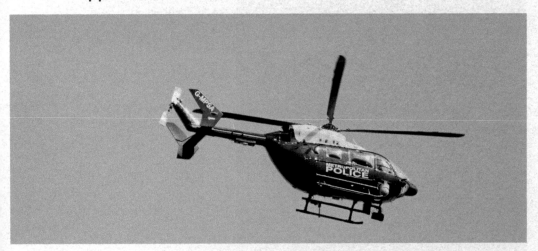

Part of the MPS Central Operations Branch, three helicopters from the National Police Air Service are based at Lippitts Hill and provide a 24-hour service to the capital. The 'all seeing eye' is able to look down all over the capital guiding officers to where they are needed most, whether it be a public order demonstration, football crowd control, major traffic congestion, vehicle pursuit or a person lost among the mass of parkland or in the water.

## Area Interceptors and Response Cars, Including Royal Parks Vehicles

The Automatic Number Plate Reading device, more commonly known as ANPR, is a comparatively new innovation, but is probably one of the most useful tools to aid policing in the fight against crime. The police driver of the unit can be automatically and instantly alerted to suspicions of any wrongdoing involving any vehicle recorded on the police database, known as PNC (Police National Computer). Area cars equipped with ANPR are marked as Interceptors. Trained to advanced police driving standards, the crew of Area cars are in addition to locally deployed Response cars – the latter dealing with all manner of general policing tasks. A selection of Response car and Royal Parks Operational Command Unit images follow, including two images in which Interceptors appear.

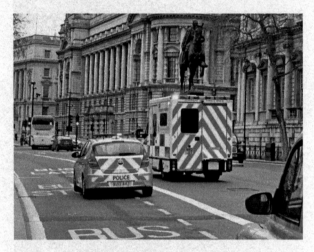

With Metropolitan Police Service (MPS) Hyundai i30 in older livery holding back its lane of traffic on Whitehall, a London Ambulance on an emergency is able to overtake in safety.

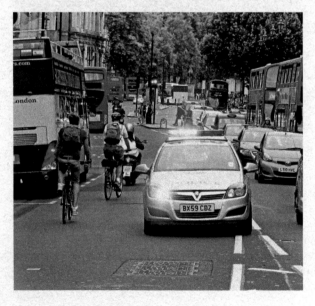

Most hours of the day the top of Whitehall is heavily congested, obliging drivers on an emergency call to go wrong side of the road in order to make progress.

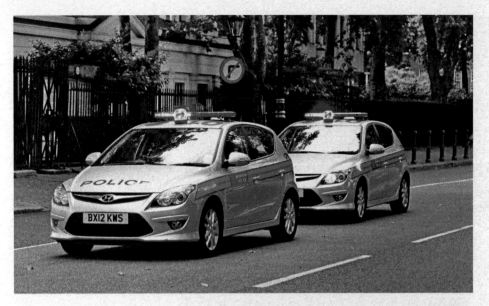

Birdcage Walk allows space in the middle of the carriageway for use in an emergency. Pictured are two parked MPS Royal Parks Operational Command Unit Hyundai i30 cars. Both vehicles are fitted with roof-mounted searchlights used at night to illuminate darkened areas of parkland.

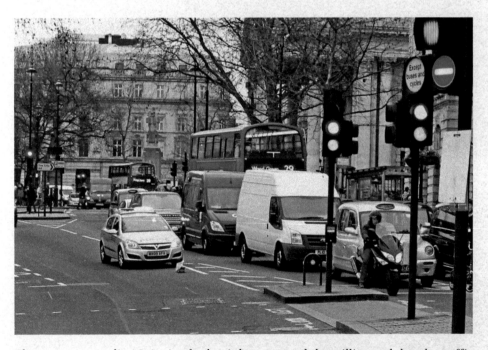

The camera never lies! It is simply that it has captured the millisecond that the traffic light sequence changes from green to amber. In the background as litter is blown across the carriageway, a Metropolitan Police Vauxhall Astra response car on an emergency is about to edge into the front of the traffic queued at Trafalgar Square's junction with Strand.

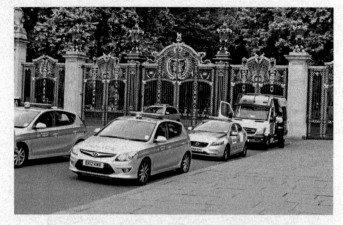

The beautiful ornate gates to Green Park provide a parking area for some of the police contingent, including a local response car, Royal Parks patrol vehicles and an Area ANPR Interceptor, all involved in the world-famous Changing of The Guard ceremony.

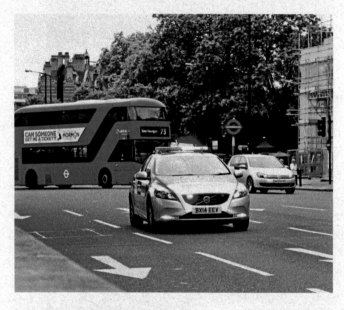

Storming around Hyde Park Corner on the blues and twos, a Volvo V40 ANPR Interceptor heads for Piccadilly.

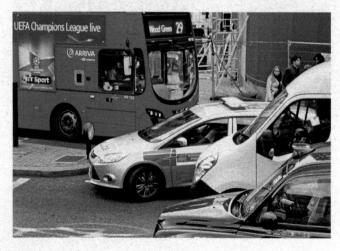

With traffic held at traffic lights adjacent to St Martin-in-the-Fields church, the local Ford Focus estate responding on an emergency is forced to come offside of the road into the path of an oncoming bus before squeezing back in.

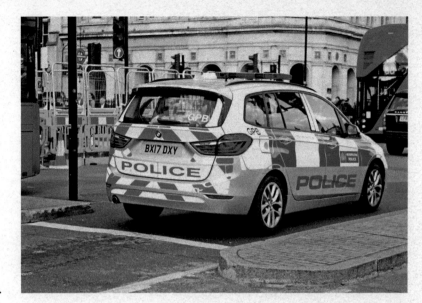

The new order in the shape of a BMW 2 series vehicle, BX17 DXY, photographed on 13 May 2017.

## Armed Response Vehicles

Responding on the blue light may appear very glamorous but for the crew they will be mindful of the enormous accountability they have for the actions they may now be about to take. On arrival at the incident, the very fact they have been tasked with responding implies they are likely to be confronted with a life-threatening situation, possibly involving the use of firearms, explosives or knives. The protection of innocent lives will be their overriding concern, no matter how dangerous the situation.

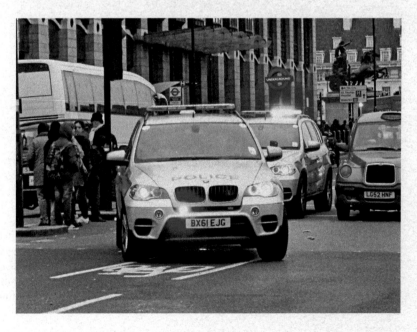

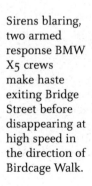

Sirens blaring, two armed response BMW X5 crews make haste exiting Bridge Street before disappearing at high speed in the direction of Birdcage Walk.

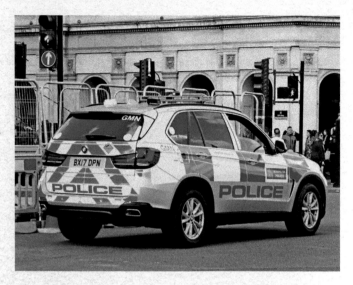

A recent BMW X5 addition to the ARV fleet, BX17 DPN makes its way towards Bridge Street.

## Cycle Patrol

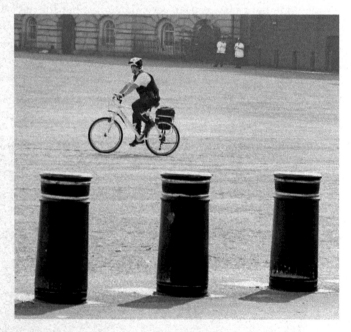

A Metropolitan Police patrolling officer having come from the St James's Park vicinity crosses the Horse Guards Parade. A Royal Parks Operational Command Unit, whose headquarters are in Hyde Park, specifically patrol many of central London's parks using cycles and vehicles. Separate Cycle Safety Teams form part of the Roads and Transport Policing Command, undertaking a vital role in driver and rider education, safety – with special regard to heavy goods vehicles, their blind spots and cyclists undertaking them – and security marking of cycles.

# Diplomatic Protection Group

The Parliamentary and Diplomatic Protection Group to give it its full title, or DPG as it is more commonly known, is responsible for the safety and security of London's diplomatic and government community. It is part of Protection Command, within the Specialist Operations directorate. To readers not familiar with London, it generally comes as a surprise to learn most of the vehicles used by this elite section are mainly red in colour.

In torrential rain, creating a curtain for the camera lens to penetrate and turning parts of the carriageway at the top of Whitehall into a river, a DPG unit responds on an emergency.

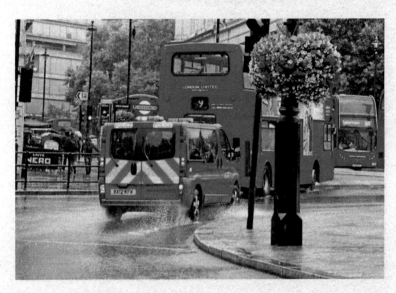

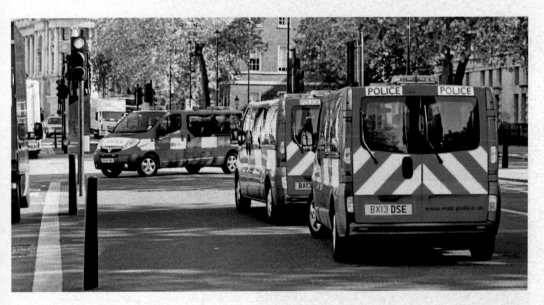

Three Vauxhall Vivaro DPG personnel carriers parked within yards of the entrance to Downing Street.

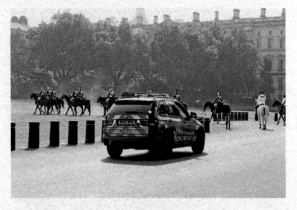

Backed up by a DPG crew in their BMW X5, mounted police officers follow members of the Household Division onto Horse Guards Parade. Some of the bollards have been lowered out of sight to grant them unimpeded access.

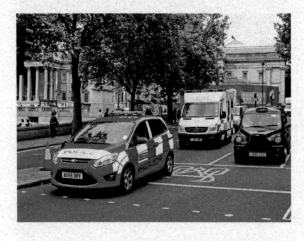

An immaculate Ford C-Max saloon is followed down the side of Trafalgar Square by an ambulance, both vehicles travelling at normal speed on separate tasks.

## Dog Support Unit

Man's best friend! Whether to maintain public order, search for explosives, drugs or for the smell of bank notes, or to track following a crime incident or missing person, the canine unit is an integral part of central London's huge daily police presence.

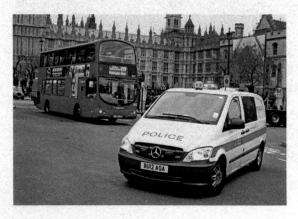

With siren wailing, a central London dog unit is about to accelerate up Whitehall on the blues.

# Foot Patrols

Times have changed and the author's days as a beat bobby in Weston-Super-Mare are not far off fifty years ago. However, I know my personal arrest rate plummeted when transferred onto Panda car patrol duties away from the back streets and lanes of the foot beat I knew so well. With it went the loss of contact with the community I served and who served me so well with friendliness and snippets of information so vital in suppressing crime and nipping problems in the bud.

Thus, it is reassuring when in central London these days to see so many uniformed officers deployed on foot, and good to see messages on social media encouraging the public to interact with them.

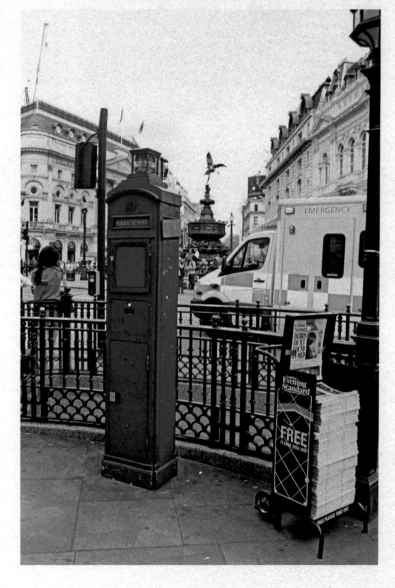

Most of this book is devoted to modern means of policing. A blast from the past can still be seen in Piccadilly Circus, overlooked by the Statue of Eros with a now obsolete public call box. It was able to give the public direct contact with the police and to allow police on foot without radios to contact their station.

# Marine Policing Unit

The MPUs role on the River Thames covers the 47 miles between Dartford and Hampton Lock, as well as responding as required to anywhere on the 250 miles of canals and other waterways in London.

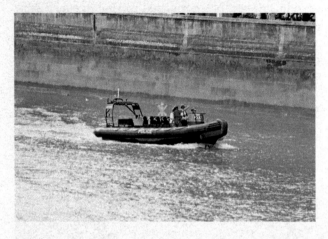

A fast response Rigid Inflatable Boat, on this occasion gently patrolling adjacent to the Houses of Parliament.

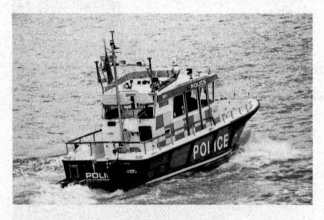

This impressive looking Targa 31, named *Gabriel Franks II,* is additionally fitted with an upper cockpit. Based at Wapping Wharf, the launch's name commemorates the first officer of the newly formed Thames River Police of 1798 to die in the line of duty, killed by rioters objecting to the force's creation.

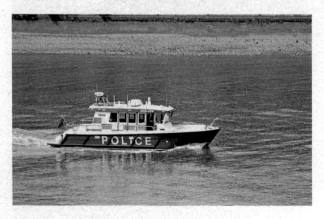

MP1, the longer Targa 37 version launch named *Patrick Colquhoun II* after the first Superintending Magistrate of the Thames River Police, makes steady progress in calm conditions at low tide.

# Mounted Branch

Another segment of the Pan London Taskforce, few sights can be more impressive than a police officer on horseback riding a magnificently groomed animal. It is very much a demanding working role, which includes traffic control and public order duties, requiring the greatest vigilance at all times, great skill, and carrying a huge weight of responsibility.

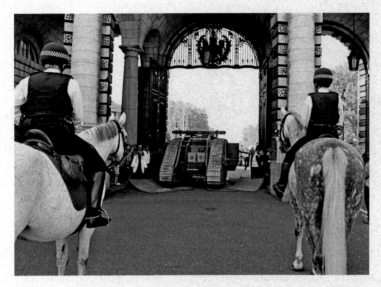

A rather unusual deployment was the provision of mounted officers to the front and rear of a replica First World War tank pictured slowly trundling through the central gateway of Admiralty Arch. The replica, used in the film *War Horse,* marked the centenary of the first use in battle on 15 September 1916 of a British tank.

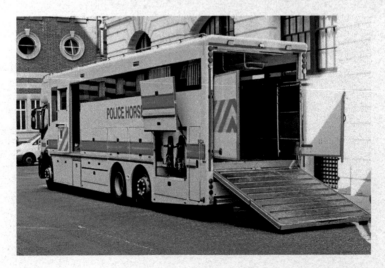

An impressive looking Iveco Stralis 330 horsebox pictured opposite the Great Scotland Yard stables.

## Police Community Support Officers

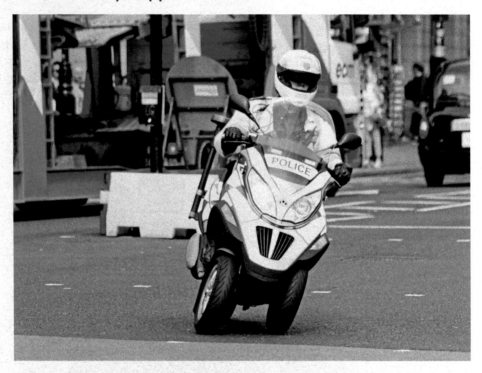

The first officers in the country were recruited by the Metropolitan Police Service in September 2002. They are a familiar sight within the capital, often seen on pedal cycle or Piaggio three-wheeled scooters equipped with extending blue light masts (as seen below).

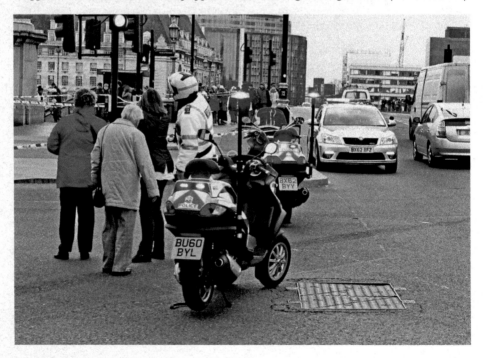

# Roads and Transport Policing Command

The Roads and Transport Policing Command are committed to reducing the number of road-related deaths and injury, as well as reducing crime, poor driving or riding standards, and driving without the necessary documentation.

Any single publication of this nature can only seek to give the reader a brief overview in both text and pictures of the vast array of vehicles – many from the Roads and Transport Policing Command – whose presence is, thankfully, continually seen on the crowded streets of central London. The deterrent effect from the presence of so many marked police vehicles and uniformed police officers can never be fully quantified but there can be no doubt they provide reassurance to the vast majority of people lawfully going about their business and help deter those with unlawful intentions.

With a huge number of cyclists using the capital each day, members work closely with Transport for London improving road safety and public transport safety. Also, working with the City of London Police they provide dedicated cycle safety teams encouraging higher standards of cycling in the capital, enforcing relevant legislation, and providing advice on cycle security. They also perform an invaluable role in helping protect cyclists by advising or reporting motorists whose actions endanger cyclists; overtaking too closely or distracted by being on a handheld phone being typical motoring offences.

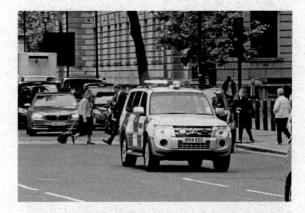

Siren helping clear the way, Mitsubishi Shogun, registration BX14 EOG, blasts its way up Whitehall on a shout.

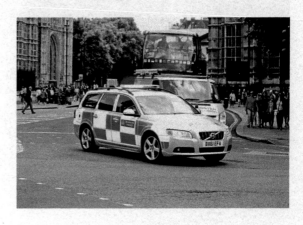

A late 2011/early 2012-registered Volvo V70 on an emergency call heads into Parliament Square from Abingdon Street.

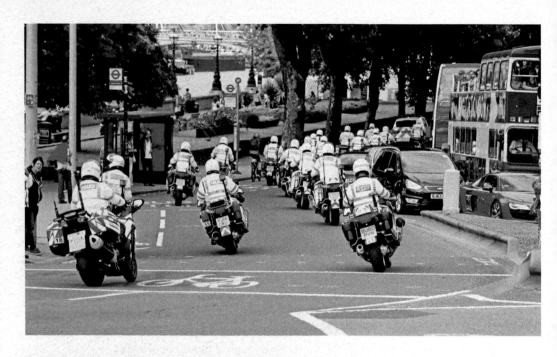

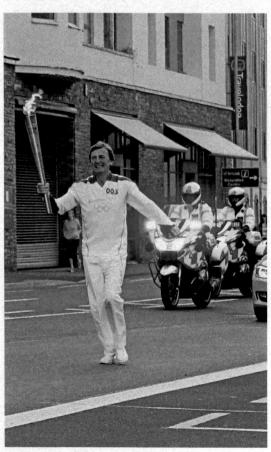

*Above*: The remarkable sight (and sound!) of approximately twenty police motorcyclists captured on camera by sheer chance; even then, one traffic car and four more motorcyclists were not in shot! They were arriving from various forces throughout the country in advance of the following day's Prudential 100-mile Ride from London through Surrey and back. This heavy contingent of police vehicles would be involved in road closures and escorting cyclists.

*Left*: With responsibility for national events crossing numerous police boundaries, Metropolitan Police runners, motorcyclists and a traffic car were instrumental in escorting 2012's Olympic Torch Relay, assisted by local officers in each force area. Just after 6 a.m. on 23 May 2012 and the torch on this short stretch is proudly held by Chris Munro from London – a significant fundraiser for MacMillan Nurses and holidays for deprived children from inner city environments. His 300-yard leg is underway in Canon's Marsh, Bristol, with Metropolitan Police motorcyclists in close proximity.

# Special Escort Group

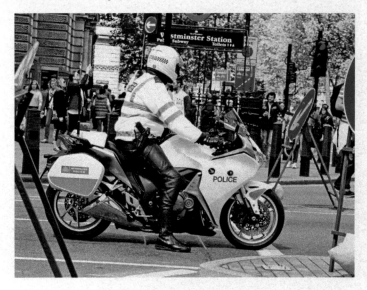

Part of the Metropolitan Police's Security Command, and instantly recognisable by their machine's distinctive registration plate and plain white livery, armed members of the SEG are a regular sight within central London. The public's attention is generally first drawn to them by the shrill blasts of their whistles – the latter a more distinctive sound to a public used to that of sirens.

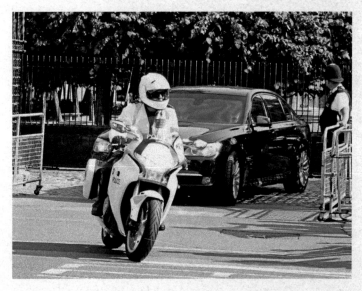

Members of the Royal family and very, very important people (VVIPs) such as the Prime Minister and visiting heads of state are escorted throughout their journeys made within the capital. One rider remains positioned at the head of the convoy, the supporting motorcyclists (the outriders) going ahead and continually leapfrogging each other in order to block approaching junctions. In this image the Prime Minister's vehicle is escorted out of the gates of the Houses of Parliament after the weekly Prime Minister's question time.

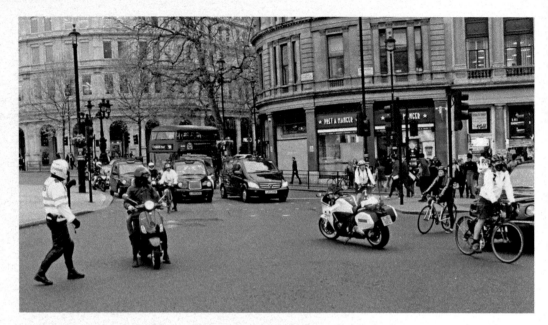

At very busy junctions an outrider is likely to rapidly dismount to undertake the very difficult task of stopping all movement, be it pedestrian or traffic including pedal cyclists. This is no easy task and it, like the entire movement, is done with a very high degree of coordination and professionalism.

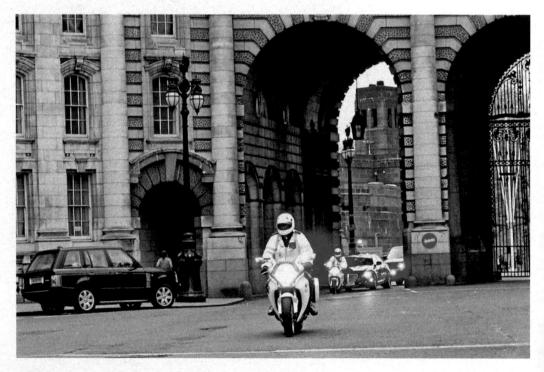

Often the wrong side of the road is used to facilitate continuous movement of the convoy, in this case the VVIP being a senior member of the Royal family.

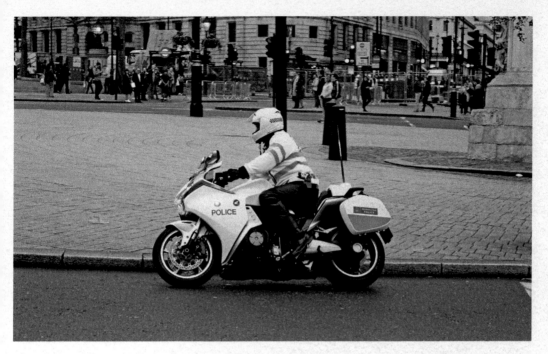

As soon as the cars pass the outrider has to rapidly remount, overtake them, and continue with fellow outriders leap frogging the junctions ahead.

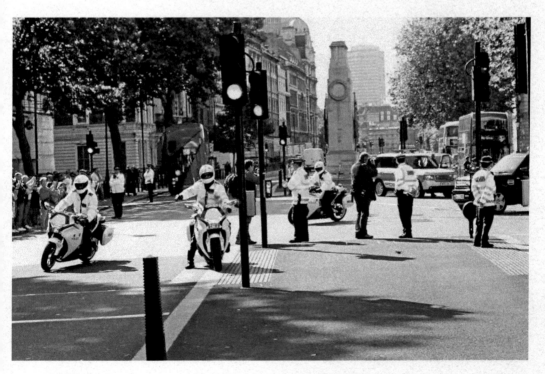

A VVIP cavalcade is pictured leaving 10 Downing Street to head wrong side of the road up Whitehall.

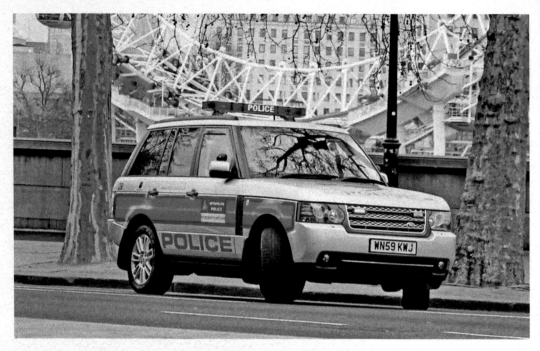

Formations may also include a marked Range Rover, which is normally positioned at the rear of the procession.

## Specialist Vehicles

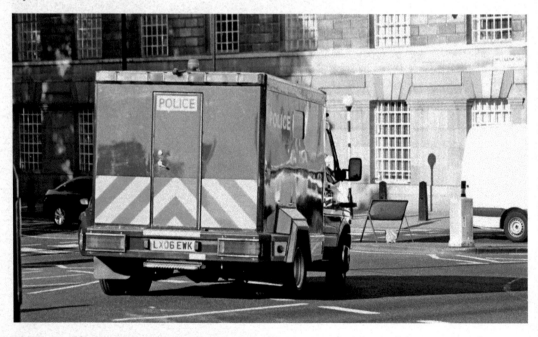

This type of high-security vehicle can sometimes be seen on television arriving at court, often as part of a high-speed police convoy.

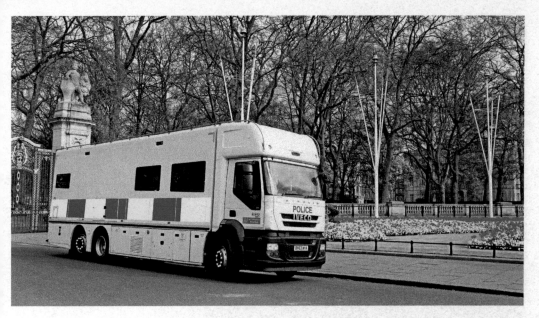

The Confined Spaces Search Team vehicle, part of the Marine Policing Unit, parked by the beautifully manicured flower bed opposite Buckingham Palace.

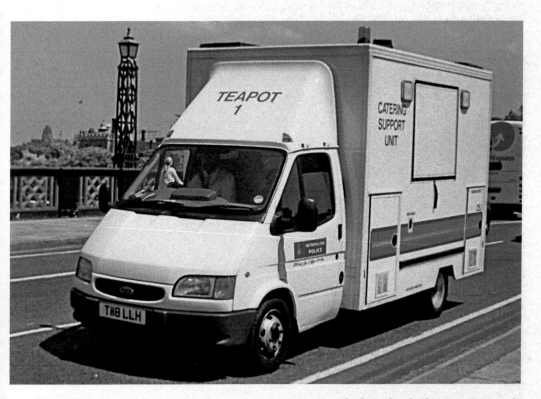

The Metropolitan Police's older 'Teapot 1', seen crossing Lambeth Bridge, had an important role to play in the organisation, providing much needed welfare facilities to the men and women on the front line at a prolonged incident.

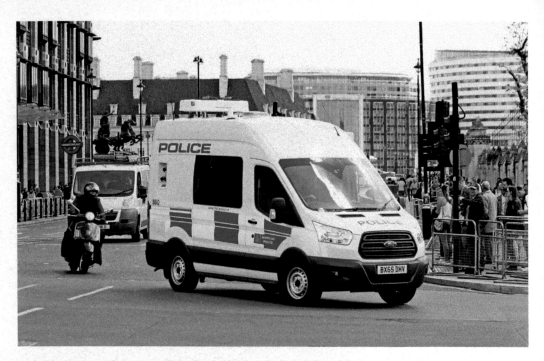

A much more modern pair of Ford vehicles has replaced the older version – this one's station code reading BBQ, the other KFC!

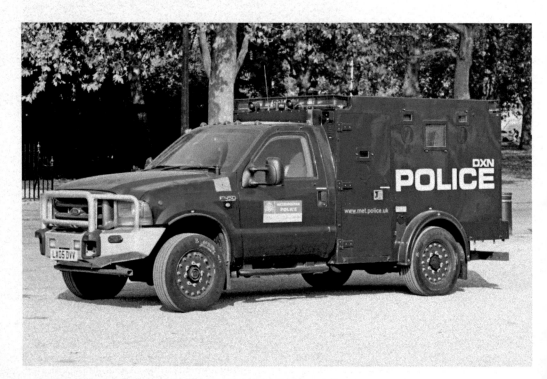

A Ford/Jankel Guardian Armoured Multi-Role Vehicle stands on a very dusty Horse Guards Parade. The majority of these heavily protected units are used on airport duties.

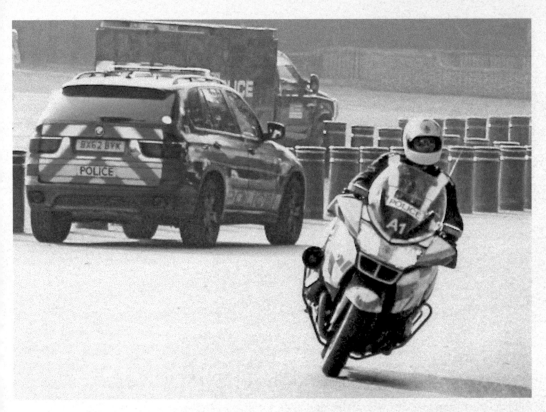

The air filled with dust rising from Horse Guards Parade after the passing of the cavalry, an impressive trio of police vehicles, including the Ford/Jankel in the background, is captured in the sweltering heat.

## Station Cell Van

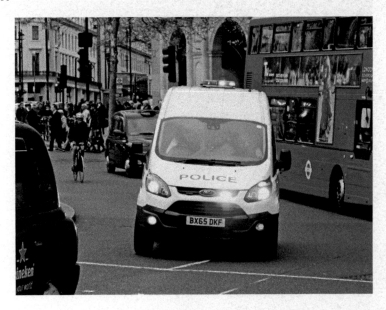

A local station van fitted with a prisoner cage in the rear responds on an emergency through Trafalgar Square.

# Territorial Support Group

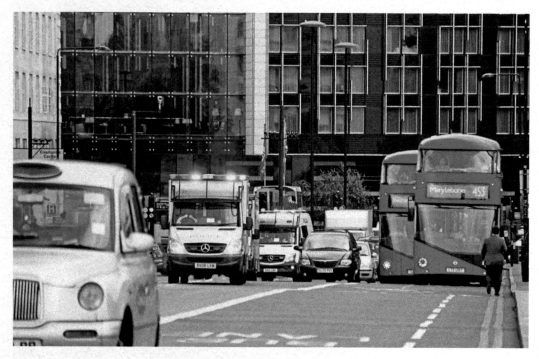

Public Order response in central London will see the attendance of Metropolitan Police Territorial Support Group (TSG) officers in their Mercedes Sprinter personnel carriers equipped with windscreen grill protection. Two older liveried vans (the second just visible) and a newer model head over Westminster Bridge in response to a call for assistance at a demonstration in Whitehall.

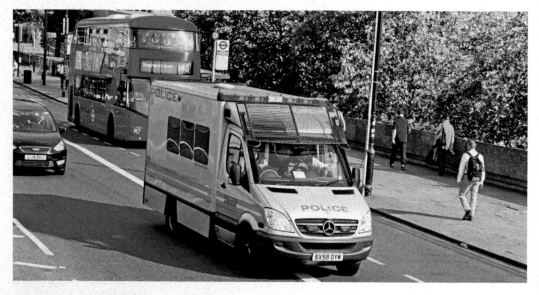

A TSG unit photographed at routine speed in central London.

# British Transport Police (BTP)

Under the command of Chief Constable Paul Crowther OBE, the force headquarters is located in Camden, London. The force has almost 3,000 police officers, 250 special constables, and over 1,500 support staff including in excess of 300 Police Community Support Officers. BTP are the national police force for the railways. In the London area this includes the national rail network, London Underground, the Docklands Light Railway, Croydon tramlink, and the Thames cable car. BTP is therefore a major player in the London policing scene with so many of the resident, business and tourist population using the above mentioned transport systems.

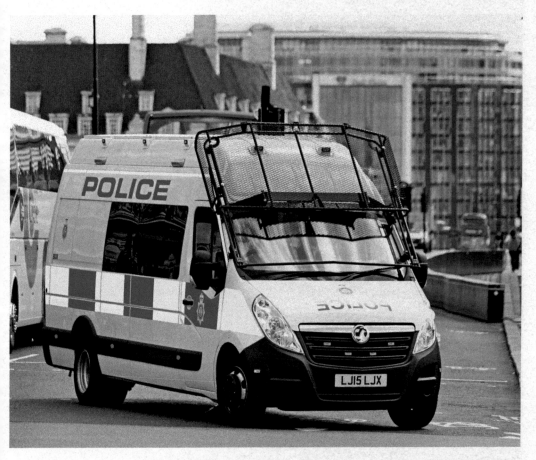

A Vauxhall Movano Police Support Unit vehicle of the type likely to be regularly deployed safeguarding the interests of travellers and railway property when large crowds pass through London's overground and underground railway network.

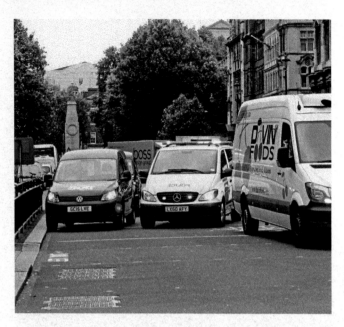

Having just performed a U-turn as a result of an emergency call being received, this BTP Mercedes Vito squeezes through the traffic.

## BTP and the Transport for London (TfL) Emergency Response Unit

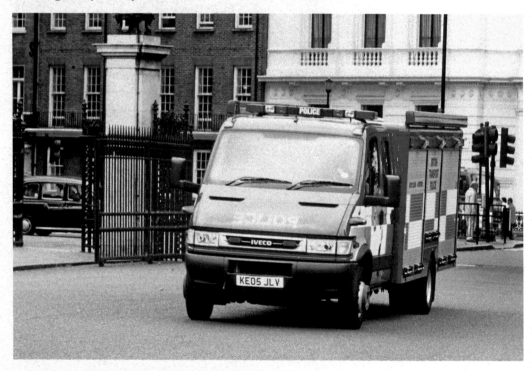

This was an earlier Iveco British Transport Police Emergency Response Unit (ERU), one of a matching pair (KE05 JLV and KE05 JLX). WX07 NWB, a Mercedes Atego ERU with police markings, was in the next generation and is now followed by the Volvos.

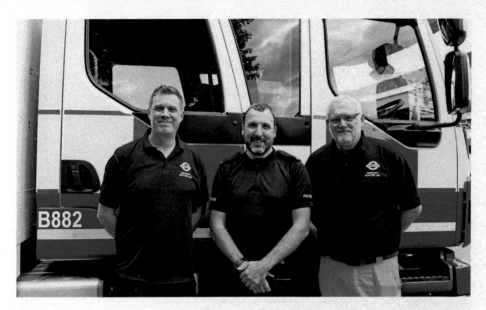

Specialist London Underground engineers Stewart Ellson (*left*) and Tony Freeman (*right*), along with BTP PC Andy Marlow (deputising with this team for PC Paul Twyman on annual leave), stood by KS66 XZW, the police-liveried Volvo FL/JDC (John Dennis Coach Builders) ERU.

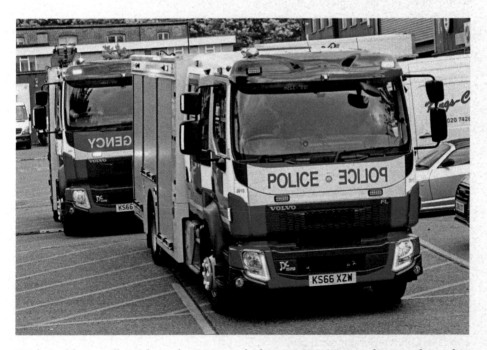

Track problems will result in the ERU marked EMERGENCY attending on the amber beacons at routine road speed. Derailment incidents will see both units attending, the police unit leading on the blues in order to facilitate the progress of both vehicles. A number of strategically positioned bases across London are equipped with similar pairs of vehicles, thus enabling multiple attendances in the more serious incidents.

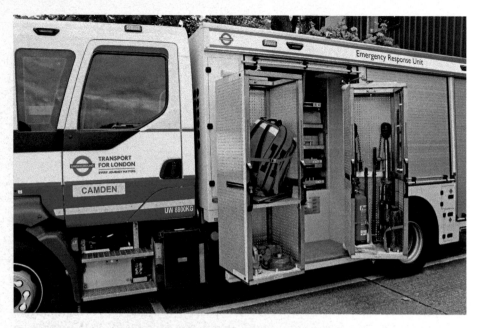

A vast array of engineering equipment is carried in the ERU marked EMERGENCY – extensive lockers supplemented by a hinged section holding even more items. The combination of BTP and LU specialist engineers attend any incident involving LU itself, London Overground, Docklands Light Railway, Tramlink networks and Network Rail operators.

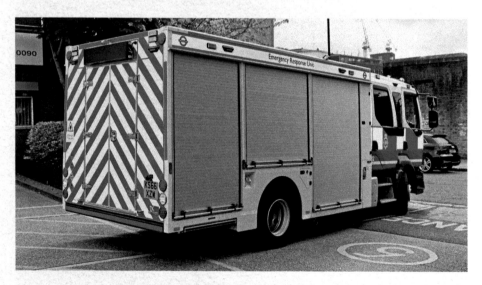

The unit marked 'POLICE' is equally well stocked with heavy equipment to assist the specialist London Underground engineers. The partnership of BTP and LU was established as a consequence of the 7 July 2005 suicide bombings that targeted London's public transport system. The ERU played a leading role supporting London's emergency services at all the affected locations in recovering the various scenes. The partnership arrangement now facilitates the early arrival at any potential life-threatening incident of the LU specialists, no matter how congested the traffic, which would otherwise hinder their progress.

# City of London Police

The 'square mile', as the City is commonly known, is the financial and economic heartland of this country as well as being a major player on the world's business stage. The City of London is a city and a county within London – the only other district of London to hold city status being adjacent Westminster. The force is commanded by Commissioner Ian Dyson QPM with headquarters in Wood Street, City. At 1,310 strong, the force has 728 sworn officers, 70 specials, and 39 PCSOs, with the remainder being civilian support staff. With a small resident population, the daily influx of business people and tourists into the City massively swells the population. The force have a very close relationship with London's other policing authorities.

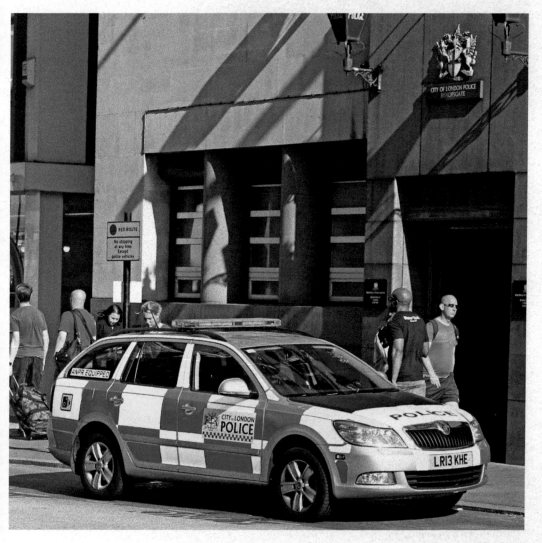

ANPR (Automatic Number Plate Reader)-equipped Skoda Octavia estate at rest outside Bishopsgate police station.

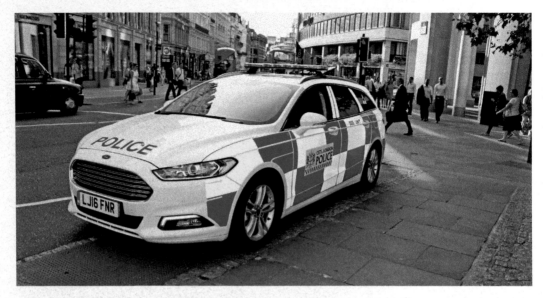

With thanks to the crews of the BMW X5 (*front cover*) and Ford Mondeo estate dog unit for permitting photography, their vehicles positioned outside St Paul's Cathedral on 13 September 2016.

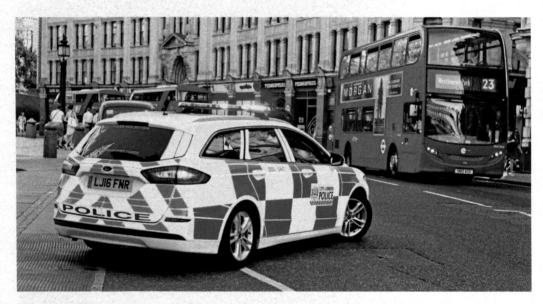

No sooner had the camera shutter been pressed for the static shots than the dog unit crew received a shout and very rapidly headed down Ludgate Hill on the blues and twos.

## Ministry of Defence Police

Commanded by Chief Constable Alf Hitchcock until he sadly passed away after a short illness, and with a strength of 2,700 officers (currently under review when preparing this section), the force is located at fifty-five establishments throughout England, Scotland and Wales.

MOD Police are not Military Police; the most obvious distinction being MOD Police wear conventional police uniform and the same badges of rank whereas Military Police wear service uniform and adhere to the military rank structure. MOD Police are responsible for policing certain government premises and the civilian elements of some military establishments.

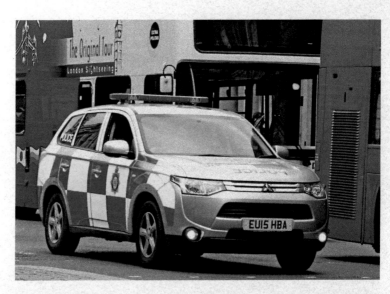

With substantial changes to vehicle propulsion likely in the coming years in a bid to create a greener environment, EU15 HBA, a Ministry of Defence Police Mitsubishi Hybrid PHEV, makes its way up Whitehall on 4 April 2017.

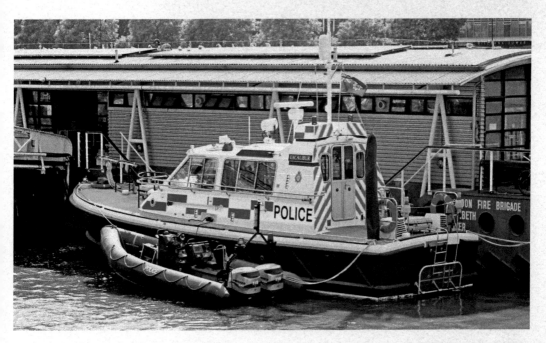

Normally based in Devonport, Plymouth, the presence of Ministry of Defence Police launch *Excalibur* seen berthed at the River fire station, Lambeth, in the summer of 2012 was probably in support of the Olympic Games security effort.

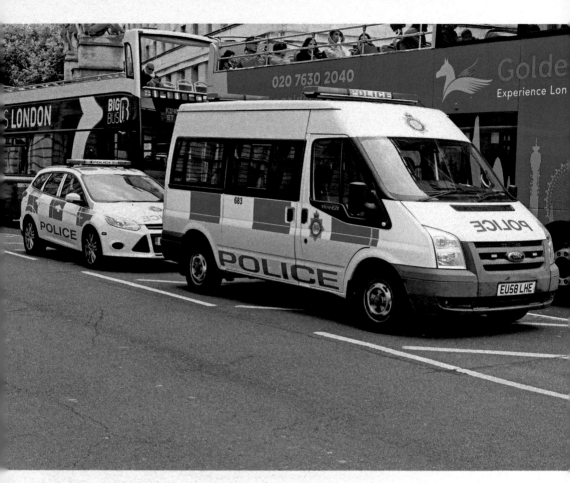

Parked adjacent to Whitehall are 2008/09-registered MOD police personnel-carrier and Ford Mondeo estate, registered EU14 FPT.

## Police National Memorial

Policing is exciting, glamorous at times, and very rewarding when officers have been able to make a positive difference to someone's life. Equally, and probably in the same shift, it can be sad, upsetting and dangerous. Stirring the sight may be as vehicles with headlights blazing and sirens blaring negotiate London's congestion, perhaps we as the public should spare a thought for the vehicle's crew, wondering where they are going and what will confront them? Almost for certain it won't be a pleasant cup of tea and biscuits; such is the nature of the job. Little was I to know as I wrote the above words in the early months of 2017, tragedy would strike at the very heart of our democracy just weeks later. Hopefully PC Palmer's family can gain some comfort from the nation's outpouring of grief, love and sympathy and from the support given to them by the serving and retired members of the Metropolitan Police Service at all levels. This very much includes the Police Family Liaison Officers and the Metropolitan Police Federation, whose dignified tweets on social media always put the interests of the family first.

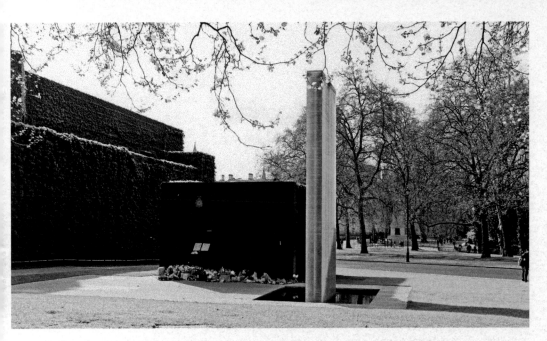

The National Police Memorial stands at the top of Horse Guards Road adjacent to The Mall. Founded in May 1984 by the late Michael Winner, the acclaimed film director, creation of The Police Memorial Trust followed the tragic death of unarmed WPC Yvonne Fletcher, who was gunned down in nearby St James's Square, Pall Mall, on 17 April 1984. Now the name of forty-eight-year-old married father, PC Keith Palmer – also simply doing his duty so that we may live in a free society – will be commemorated forever more both here and in an individual memorial adjacent to the spot where he fell in New Palace Yard, part of the Palace of Westminster. May he rest in peace.

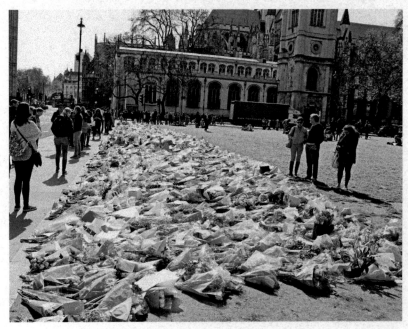

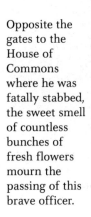

Opposite the gates to the House of Commons where he was fatally stabbed, the sweet smell of countless bunches of fresh flowers mourn the passing of this brave officer.

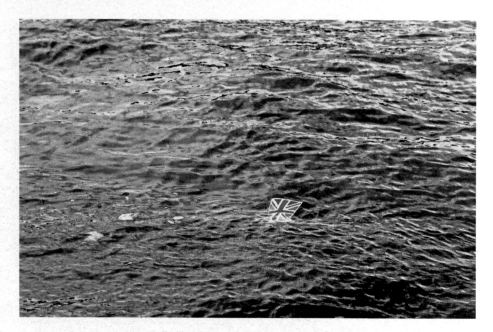

Terrorists hitting London, and on 22 May 2017, Manchester, killing twenty-three innocent people including off-duty Cheshire policewoman Elaine McIver, may try to sink the British spirit. The resolve of our emergency services – the likes of the gentleman in the next image – and the determination of the overwhelming majority of the British public will ensure that never happens.

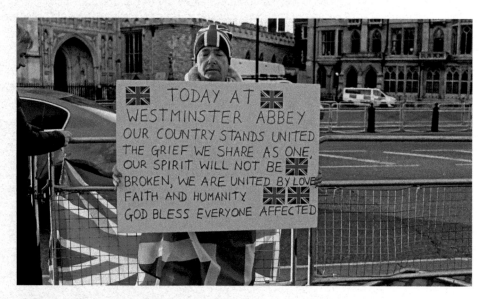

7.14 a.m. 5 April 2017 opposite Westminster Abbey, a few early arrivals start to assemble in readiness to witness the gathering of so many involved in the tragic events of 22 March 2017 in the Service of Hope, led by royalty, starting at noon. No words of mine can match these. I can only echo the sentiments expressed on the board this gentleman had composed. His sincerity was equally matched by his spoken word in the few minutes I was privileged to spend chatting with him.

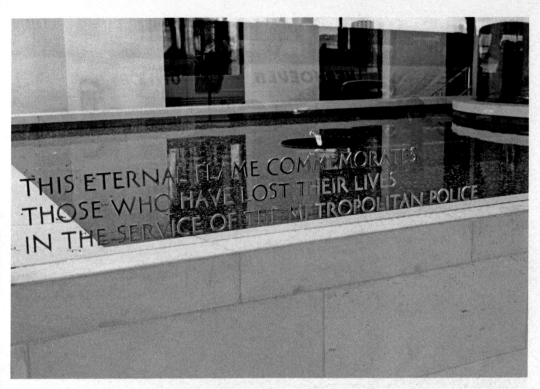

The Eternal Flame poignantly glows behind its glass screen at New Scotland Yard on Victoria Embankment.

THIS ETERNAL FLAME COMMEMORATES
THOSE WHO HAVE LOST THEIR LIVES
IN THE SERVICE OF THE METROPOLITAN POLICE.

May you, PC Keith Palmer, posthumously awarded the George Medal for bravery, and those who have fallen before, and all your families, be forever in our minds and hearts.

# CHAPTER 4

# Royal National Lifeboat Institution

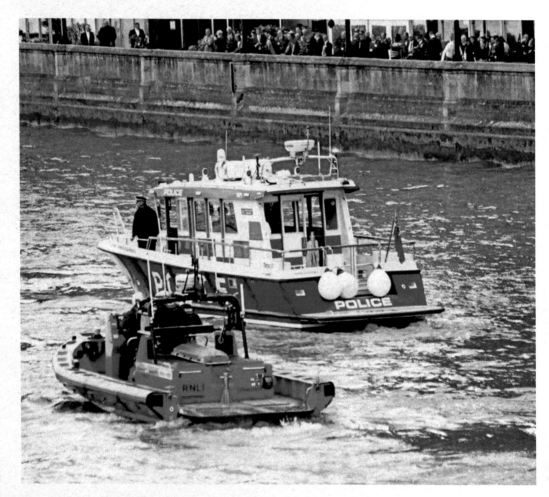

RNLI E-class lifeboat E-07 *Hurley Burly* alongside Metropolitan Police launch, MP1, *Patrick Colquhoun II.*

# Introduction

Following the disaster of 20 August 1989, when the dredger *Bowbelle* collided with the pleasure vessel *Marchioness,* causing the loss of fifty-one lives, in 2002 the RNLI took over the primary role of search and rescue on the River Thames. Four lifeboat stations were established at Gravesend, Tower Pier, Chiswick Pier and Teddington. In 2006 the Tower Pier operation transferred to Waterloo Pier to cover the central part of London, retaining the name Tower lifeboat station. Now well established as the busiest station in the RNLI, for the year 2016 this station's vessels were launched 512 times, rescuing 72 people, and saving 19 lives. *Hurley Burly* based there is a vessel specifically designed for the River Thames. It is a fast response, waterjet powered, inshore E-class lifeboat operating exclusively within the tidal reach of the River Thames.

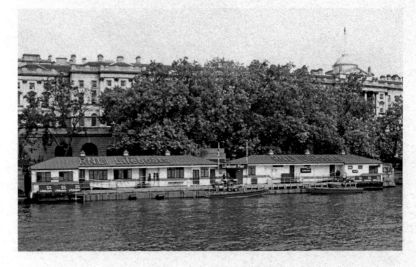

Formerly a Metropolitan Police Marine Police base located just below Waterloo Bridge, the RNLI's Tower lifeboat station now occupies the structure.

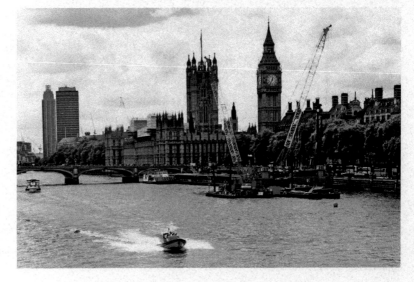

From a speck in the distance just seconds beforehand, it was not long before the high-speed craft, travelling at around its maximum speed of 40 knots (46 mph), became recognisable as the inshore lifeboat.

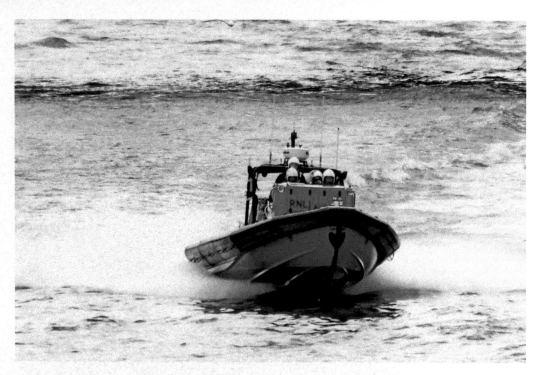

Crew suitably kitted, this extremely fast craft was rapidly in attendance at a reported incident near Hungerford Bridge.

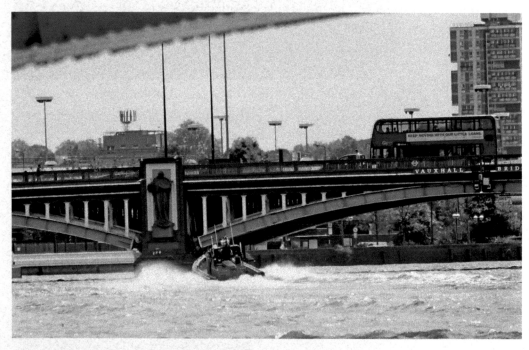

A long-range lens captures *Hurley Burly* on a separate mission, thrashing the waves as she approaches Vauxhall Bridge at high speed; a person had been spotted in the river.

# Conclusion

## Supporting the Front Line

A myriad of workers behind the scenes ensure London's emergency services can function effectively, efficiently, and as economically as possible – their roles too diverse to mention individually, but to whom a deep debt of gratitude is owed.

Major incidents are very rare, yet London has been hit by an unprecedented three within the same number of months. Since copy material for this book went to the publishers subsequent to the Westminster Bridge incident of 22 March 2017, there has been the London Bridge and nearby Borough Market, Southwark, terrorist incident of 3 June 2017, with eight people murdered and forty-eight injured by a trio of terrorists shot dead at the incident by police. The massive fire at the Grenfell Tower residential block, Latimer Road, North Kensington, occurred just before 1 a.m. on 14 June 2017, claiming the lives of eighty residents – as per the official number at the time of writing – and injuring many more. Sixty-three people were rescued by extremely brave firefighters from the London Fire Brigade. The twenty-four-storey building of 120 flats was almost completely gutted in a rapid and unprecedented fire spread, and the incident is now the subject of a public inquiry.

## Control Room Staff

No emergency service can function without those largely unsung heroes in the respective control room or operations centre. They are the individuals receiving the emergency calls, making sense of what distraught callers are saying, and mobilising the appropriate resources. The public's lives are as much in their hands, especially in the initial stages of the incident, as they are in the hands of those attending to resolve the emergency.

## The Text

The objective of this book has been to provide a vivid and up-to-date pictorial record as of early 2017 of the diverse range of emergency services vehicles to be seen in the last few years in central London. It was never to provide reams of historical, organisational or technical information; that is left to others more qualified to do so. Nevertheless, it is hoped the information in relation to the services featured, no matter how brief, will have been of interest.

## The Images

The wide range of images has taken numerous visits to the capital and countless hours to try and capture. Despite various limitations, a reasonable cross-section has made it into the pages of this book. I hope you find as much enjoyment in looking at these images as I have from the challenge of photographing them.

## All Emergency Service Personnel

The emergency services activity represented through the medium of the camera is very much part of the reality of daily life in central London.

To all crews and staff behind the scenes, no matter what emergency service they represent, and whether salaried staff or volunteers, the public should be grateful. Fortunately, the vast majority of the population are supportive, understanding and appreciative of what our emergency services do. Long may that continue!

## Donations

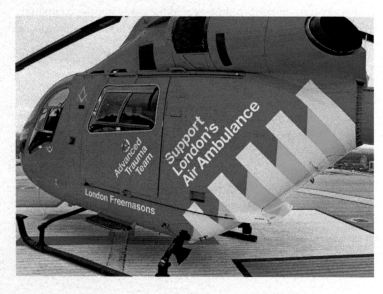

This vital aid to the saving of life was funded by £4 million of donations.

Organisations such as the British Red Cross Society, London's Air Ambulance Charity (and similar air ambulance organisations throughout the country), the Royal National Lifeboat Institution, the Salvation Army (who provide catering facilities to London Fire Brigade at major incidents), and St John Ambulance are largely funded by charitable donations. Should you be minded to make any donation, it will, no matter how small, be greatly appreciated by the relevant organisation.

## Thanks

Thanks are due to: Tim Ash, Press & Public Relations Officer, Royal National Lifeboat Institution; London; Lloyd Buckingham for his IT assistance; Watch Manager Mike Cotton, London Fire Brigade – fire officer and fire appliance preservationist; prolific transport author and good friend Martin S. Curtis for his encouragement in seeking to have this work published; Inspector Stuart Downs and PC Andy Marlow of British Transport Police, along with Stewart Ellson and Tony Freeman of Transport for London's London Underground Emergency Response Unit; vehicle historian and photographer Matt Holmes for his friendship over many years; Watch Manager Tony Marshall and Firefighter Keiron Maden at Euston fire station; Alan Matthews, chairman of the Police Vehicle Enthusiasts Club; NHS Blood & Transplant (National Organ Retrieval Service), Stoke Gifford, Bristol; the Royal London Hospital; Personnel at Dowgate, Euston, Paddington and Soho fire stations; Alexandra Sutherland, Media and Public Affairs Officer and Paul Smith, Helipad Manager, both of London's Air Ambulance Charity; The Tank Museum, Bovington, Dorset; and especially to my wife Margaret for her skill with the camera and help in compiling this book.

## The Author

Dave's main career was in the police service, serving with Avon & Somerset Constabulary for ten years and then the Ministry of Defence Police until retiring in 1996, having reached the rank of chief superintendent. In 2000 he became the regional accident investigator for FIRST Bus. Adopting the attitude of trying to prevent accidents happening, he designed and presented a successful accident prevention course, before carrying on his efforts to reduce the blameworthy accident rate among bus and coach drivers during a period of self-employment. For his successful endeavours he was honoured with the MBE in 2007. During the 2016/17 winter he turned his hand to writing, combining this with his lifelong passion for both the emergency services and photography to produce this, his first work.

# Sources

## Twitter

Numerous daily tweets over several years from a mass of contributors.

## Websites of

British Transport Police
City of London Police
London's Air Ambulance Charity
London Ambulance Service
London Fire and Emergency Planning Authority
Metropolitan Police Service
Ministry of Defence Police
Royal National Lifeboat Institution

## Dedication

With the emergency services in the family blood over several generations, some twenty-five years ago I vowed to produce a photographic record of the 999 services for any grandchildren I was eventually blessed with so they could have a permanent record for their own families to come, thus passing on my knowledge to future generations.

Therefore, it is with very real pleasure I dedicate this book not only to my daughters Anna and Sue, and son-in-law John, but to grandchildren Holly, Jamie, Lewis, Finley, Amber, Ruby and Erin.

Dave Boulter MBE
Yate, South Gloucestershire
12 July 2017